GEROETHICS

Golden Age Books

Perspectives on Aging

Series Editor: Steven L. Mitchell

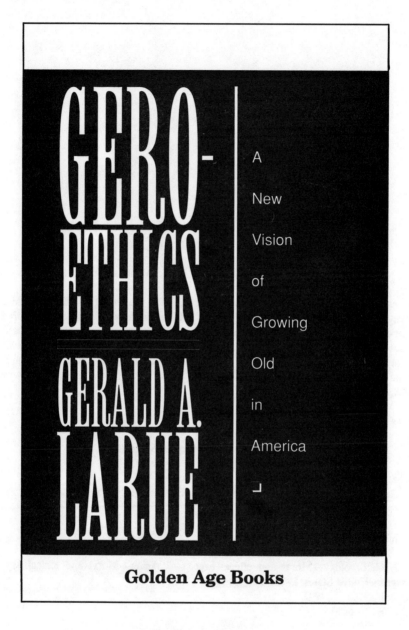

GERO-ETHICS

A New Vision of Growing Old in America

GERALD A. LARUE

Golden Age Books

Prometheus Books

59 John Glenn Dr., Buffalo, NY 14228-2197

Published 1992 by Prometheus Books

96 95 94 93 92   5 4 3 2 1

Library of Congress Cataloging-in-Publication Data

Larue, Gerald A.
    Geroethics : a new vision of growing old in America / by Gerald A. Larue.
        p.   cm.—(Golden age books)

    Includes bibliographical references
    ISBN 0-87975-750-7 (cloth)
    1. Gerontology—Moral and ethical aspects. 2 Aging—Moral and ethical aspects.
3. Aged—United States. I. Title. II. Series.
HQ1061.L3565   1992
305.26′0973—dc20   92-15264
                                                                 CIP

Printed in the United States of America on acid-free paper.

Dedication

To Audrey and Frances, Paul and Bud, wonderful elders who may bend but refuse to bow to the infirmities of old age and who, together with those who love them, live full and meaning-filled lives.

Contents

10   Contents

Preface

This book has had a long history. Its roots go back to the courses that I taught during the summer sessions at the Andrus Center nearly fifteen years ago. During those early years, I was privileged to meet an amazing group of men and women from many parts of the world from whom I learned and with whom I shared insights that had grown out of my studies of ancient Near Eastern life and literature. Ethical issues from the ancient past echo in society's present-day concerns. Subsequently, after retirement from the School of Religion, I became a member of the teaching staff at the center. One of my courses dealt with value issues and aging.

In 1989, I was recognized by the American Humanist Society as "Humanist of the Year," an honor that was completely unexpected and which placed me on a list with former honorees that included some of the finest scientists and thinkers in the world. My acceptance speech was titled "Geroethics." In 1990, I was invited to participate in a National Long-Term Care conference in Calgary, Alberta, Canada, sponsored by the Alberta Long-Term Care Association. Once again I focused on "Geroethics." Obviously it was time for a book.

Special credit must be given to some of my recent students in the Leonard Davis School of Gerontology at the Andrus Center, University of Southern California. These dedicated young men and women who are preparing to enter the work force as gerontologists, geriatricians, or other professionals linked to aging, produced excellent research papers that challenged my thinking and called my attention to important source materials. Some of their ideas have been incorporated in this book. I thank them and I list some of their names: Thomas X. C. Cuyegkeng, Father

13

Richard Erikson, Holly Fleischman, Debbie Fox, Xiaohua Jiang (Beijing), Marti Klein, Christopher Kuhar, Meng-Fan Li (Taiwan), Robert Larriva, Ernesto Paredes, Shauna L. Reel, Jenny Shin, and Shannon Poth Ward.

Gerald Moyer of the Los Angeles County Social Work Department opened important doors for me with the invitation to meet with Los Angeles County Social Workers to discuss elder abuse. These wonderful, dedicated persons who work in some of the most dangerous and depressing environments not only gave me the opportunity to share my deepest concerns, but responded with insights developed out of experience, all of which enhanced my growth. In addition, Gerald Moyer provided me with the excellent materials produced by the county to instruct and guide elders and case workers. I cannot find adequate words to express my admiration and appreciation for these fine, overworked, and underpaid persons. They may recognize some of their responses in the section of this book dealing with elder abuse.

Once again, it has been my privilege to work with my editor and friend, Steven L. Mitchell. Our association goes back many years to our association with the Academy of Humanism, but this year has been particularly enriched through the publishing of two books, one a collection of essays dealing with long-term care and this present volume. As always, the publisher of Prometheus Books, Dr. Paul Kurtz, a long-time friend and colleague whom I admire and care about more than I can articulate, has been a behind-the-scenes supporter of this publication.

The names listed in the dedication represent persons who have been part of me for most of my life. They are my brothers and sisters who continue to amaze me with their courage and the differing ways by which they handle the vicissitudes of age. They, their spouses, and their children form an important part of my inner circle of love and respect. Finally, I cannot fail to thank my wife, Emily Perkins Larue, whose love and caring sustains me more than she can know.

1

What Is "Geroethics"?

"If we can leave our humanity aside for a moment and put our human sense of values out of mind, we must admit that the world is neither good nor evil, that such categories do not apply to the life of a butterfly or a crab. It is, however, another matter when we are dealing with our own demands, demands peculiar to us amid everything alive."

—Czeslaw Milosz, *Visions from San Francisco Bay,* p. 174

For many, elders are shadow people. They are there but are only dimly part of the current scene. They become briefly recognizable when someone complains about the "little old man" or "little old lady" who, while driving on the freeway at the posted 55 miles an hour, is holding up traffic because everyone else wants to go faster. At the supermarket between 1:30 and 3:00 P.M., elders are often seen pushing their shopping carts up and down the aisles, sometimes talking with the cashier who takes time to inquire about their grandchildren and to ask how they are feeling. Patrons who get in line behind them may sigh with impatience as they open their coin purses to fumble for the correct change to pay for their one banana, one cup of cottage cheese, one tomato, and perhaps a can of cat food. They come every day about the same time, follow the same routine, speak to the same cashiers, and converse with one another before going on their way. They are the elders, the shadow people, who manifest themselves briefly before they disappear.

Who is that wizened old oriental with the chest cough? Who knows that he speaks four languages—Vietnamese, Chinese, French, and English— or that when the Vietnam war broke out he fled from the Communist north to the south where he worked with Americans? Who knows that seven years ago he, with his wife and four sons, joined some 700 other Vietnamese refugee boat people to seek asylum elsewhere? They lived in their overcrowded boat for weeks, subsisting on rice and other staples, including the huge white Asian radishes that assuaged their thirst as they were refused entry at Singapore, and then at other ports until they came to Indonesia. Who knows of their struggle to come to America and of the hard work and long hours needed to be self-supporting, free citizens? Who cares about a shadowy little oriental, or indeed about any other elder one meets on the street? Of what importance are they or their stories?

Elders are not to be categorized along with the crab or the butterfly as existing in a world where neither good nor evil apply. They are important because they are, in so many ways, involved in dealing with "our own demands, demands peculiar to us amid everything else alive." They are more than shadow people; they are part of us, and ethical values are issues as important and vital to them as they are to the rest of society.

Geroethics is the consideration of ethical principles with regard to a particular segment of the population: the elders. Ethics can be defined as the study of moral principles that provide guides for individual or societal life, including standards of conduct and regulations concerning what is right and wrong and what constitutes moral duties and obligations. Within given disciplines or professions, ethical standards outline rules for determining acceptable conduct. Ethical principles embrace concepts of rights and privileges, duties and obligations, choices and their results. Geroethics seeks to consider the ways in which societal values impact on elders and how the aged may respond to these same values.

WHO MAKES THE RULES?

The rules, regulations, or principles that guide the choices of any particular group of people develop out of community, out of humans living together. When situations arise requiring the making of decisions affecting societal well-being, the choices made by the group are either fair or unfair, just or unjust, decent or indecent, life-enhancing or life-inhibiting. As those choices crystalize and become codified, they form the basic ethic of a group, a community, or a nation. Subsequently, acts are judged to be good or bad, moral or immoral, nourishing or toxic on the basis of conformity to accepted ethical standards.

The ethics adopted or developed by a society describes its value system indicating what is considered to be of worth or significance and what is of little or no worth in the eyes of the group. These accepted values or beliefs, customs or institutions, assume power in and of themselves to arouse emotional responses in a given society, group, or individual. To value is to make a choice and to act upon that choice. For the individual and for the society, the choices made and the acts they occasion reflect the moral core of societal or personal history. The value choices and acts also represent the results of a search for that which gives meaning to life.

Personal values usually reflect the individual's societal environment. In one way or another, either subtly or forthrightly, each group projects concepts of acceptable social attitudes. These may include beliefs and feelings about slavery, or the inferiority of certain races, places of origin, religions, and so forth. A child's family instills values that may emphasize honesty and diligence or may produce bigotry and phobias. Institutions impact on the developing person. The school may stress fair play, the importance of making decisions on the basis of factual knowledge, and self-reliance as opposed to dependence on cheating. Religious institutions may emphasize the importance of love, humility, peace, and so forth. In other words, an individual's moral code and behavior will be the result of a melding of input from a number of societal sources plus the person's thoughtful evaluation of what he or she is being taught. The value system developed by the individual, like that of society in general, may be judged to be ethical or unethical on the basis of how it ennobles the person and how it limits or enhances the rights and privileges of others.

Basic to our survival are the requirements of food, clothing, shelter and community. How these needs are met and satisfied involves choices that affect the self and others in either positive or negative ways. Almost every culture has laws prohibiting theft, deceit, murder, and the like. The concern is for social "justice," however defined. The so-called Golden Rule recognizes the individual as a choice maker and acknowledges the effect of choices on others. The idea of doing to others what you would have them do to you or, in the negative form, not doing to others what you would not want them to do to you, is almost universal. One may prefer what Barrows Dunham (1971) has called "the more rigorous Kantian version 'Treat everyone, yourself included, as an end; never treat anyone merely as a means.' " He points out that "this rule, applied, will shape decisions and their consequences, but it will also create a proper climate of decision" (ibid). Obviously, such precepts developed out of the need for guidelines for successful and reasonable living together. They are humanistic principles, not divinely revealed, although some societies give the Golden Rule the authority of a deity. These and similar notions provide a basis for regulations against stealing, lying, physical abuse, and so on and beliefs about the importance of human worth, human freedom, dignity, justice, and the like. Those principles that appear to be positive or nourishing and life-enhancing are often labelled "good," while those that are toxic and life-denying are viewed as "evil."

Of course, in some societies ethical prescriptions do not embrace everyone; freedom to make choices is deemed to be the prerogative of a dominant group. Ignoring the rights of minorities results in unfair treatment and enslavement of a group (such as African-Americans) or violence because of a belief system (such as in the persecution of witches) or subordination on the basis of sex (as represented in the role of women in Saudi Arabia). As awareness of universal human rights develops, dehumanizing and freedom-limiting rules change. African-Americans, no longer slaves, are slowly breaking down the social barriers that still limit their achievement of full human rights to employment, education, justice, and so on. Persecution of witches belongs to the past as a testimony to a sorry and sick religious ethic. Some women in Saudi Arabia are beginning to express dissatisfaction with their limited social status. In other words, ethical principles, whether or not they are endorsed by church and state, can be toxic and evil, but they can be changed by pressure from those whose vision of social and ethical norms embraces all humans regardless of race or creed, color or sex, wealth or age. The highest ethic seeks to validate the full humanity of all persons, guaranteeing for all equal rights to the benefits of society and to the opportunities to fulfill themselves as persons insofar as the execution of those rights do not interfere with or hinder the opportunities and rights of others.

RULE ETHICS AND SITUATION ETHICS

One can accept a set of rules as ethically binding and apply these to each and every situation, or one can recognize the regulations as guidelines that can be affected by the uniqueness of a situation. The conflict between "rule ethics" and "situation ethics" (as set forth by Joseph Fletcher) has been recognized and debated (Fletcher 1966, pp. 11–13). Those who follow a rule ethic have decisions made *a priori:* the "choice is dictated by rule" (Fletcher 1979, p. 3). The unique factors in a setting are irrelevant because the decision is already formulated. According to Fletcher, "The fundamental ethical question is whether we are to live and act by rules or by reason . . . it is wiser to be guided by moral principles than by moral rules" (1979, p. 5). As he has noted, "In a free society we have no official ethics any more than we have an official faith or political philosophy. But we can have a moral consensus" (1966, pp. 158–59). This moral consensus forms the basis for much of the discussion in this book.

ETHICS AND GEROETHICS

Geroethics, therefore, focuses on ethical principles as they apply to elders. Perhaps the basic ethical concerns are no different from those pertaining to any other age group, but the ways in which fundamental values relate to elders and the ways in which elders relate to these values have unique dimensions or colorations. For example, the right to choose to live or die may have quite different implications for a thirty-year-old and someone fifty years older. Problems of survival may have separate meanings for elders and teenagers. Yet, the ethical principles are similar and related.

In this volume I try to evaluate, in terms of ethics, what is happening in the expanding society of elders. How do accepted ethical principles or guidelines affect the lives of the graying generation? I begin by trying to determine just who and what are the elders (who include persons born during the first quarter of this twentieth century and who are now sixty-five years of age or older). Then I focus briefly on the value systems that underlie the concept of citizenship before turning to issues of "survival" and "meaning" for elders. My concern is with the raising of consciousness regarding geroethics both today and for the future when the numbers of elders will double and triple. The problems confronting the present generation of elders foreshadows difficulties that will confront future elders, which, if they are not properly solved now, will be waiting for the upcoming generations as they enter the ranks of the elderly. Finding solutions to geroethical problems is the responsibility of everyone and in the best interests of us all.

"ELDERS"?

Perhaps the choice of the label "elder" needs some explanation. Like so many, I am wearied by descriptive labels such as "gray heads," "old people," and "the aged," each of which conjures up a mental image that can be denigrating. My daughter-in-law calls me "Senior" to avoid confusion because her husband and her son are named after me. I like the term because it signifies a familial relationship, but when applied to a population of older persons, it really conveys little or nothing. The term "elder" relates not only to age but also to status based both on age and experience. In some religious communities it signifies a position of standing; in simpler societies it bears overtones of accumulated wisdom. Hence, for our purposes, "elder" signifies age, experience, status, and, in most instances, wisdom.

REFERENCES

Dunham, Barrows. 1971. *Ethics Dead and Alive*. New York: Alfred A. Knopf, Inc.

Fletcher, Joseph. 1966, *Situation Ethics*. Philadelphia: The Westminster Press.

———. 1979. *Humanhood: Essays in Biomedical Ethics*. Buffalo, N.Y.: Prometheus Books.

Larue, Gerald, A. 1980. "Geroethics: A Humanist Issue," *The Humanist* 49, no. 4 (July-August): 5–10, 38.

Milosz, Czeslaw. 1982. *Visions from San Francisco Bay*. Translated by Richard Lourie. New York: Farrar Strauss Giroux.

2

The Elders: Who Are They?

"For we who have lived half a century or more have already enjoyed a very interesting and varied existence with probably a good deal of personal happiness. . . . And if in my remaining years I can make a worthwhile contribution to society, I shall be happy indeed."

—Corliss Lamont, *Yes to Life,* p. 205

Who are the elders? How do we define them? Do we visualize them as a group or a collection of groups? Are they to be recognized as beneficial contributors to society or as benign artifacts neither contributing nor detracting but just existing, or as detrimental drains on national resources giving nothing in return for what they receive? How we perceive elders reflects the true value we place on them and determines our ethical response.

We think about aging in different ways. For some people aging simply means growing old or becoming aged. On the basis of this definition, studies in geriatric medicine and in gerontology focus on old people and their needs, ranging from the physical through the social, psychological, environmental, economic and on through other such dimensions. Another way of looking at aging is developmentally or in terms of growth or maturation cycles. References are made to the stages (Shakespeare called them "ages") through which humans progress. Theorists and developmental psychologists inform us that as we move from one particular "age" into the next in the life cycle, we do not abandon or leave behind the influences and implications of former stages of development. Some would argue that we do not successfully enter into a new stage without having completed

21

the inherent developmental patterns of the present stage. This way of thinking about aging tends to lock individuals into strictly labelled age-groups as being at a particular "stage" of development (see chapter 4 on "Agism"). I tend to avoid such categorizations, except where I feel the final "stage" may provide some insight into the role and significance of elders.

For our purposes, aging refers to the normal, natural process of change and maturation that is incorporated into the genetic structure (DNA) of every living thing. Life is a process involving development that, according to some, begins at the moment of fertilization but in this discussion is thought to start at birth when the infant has, for the first time, evolved (i.e., left the vulva) as an independent entity, breathing and eating, and existing separate from the mother. The newborn comes equipped with inherited genetic patterns that can determine everything from reactions to certain substances to tendencies to acquire certain illnesses. The infant has already been affected by the diet of the mother, whether or not she used drugs, the quality of the air she breathed and the amount of toxic waste that might be deposited in the soil beneath the home in which she has lived. We do not enter the world unaffected by what has taken place during the nine months prior to birth. Nevertheless, our independent life begins at birth when we first start to adjust to the world as separate living beings.

The developmental or maturation process of the individual continues from birth to the moment of death when all growth, all development, all change ceases. For some organisms, such as insects, the process is rapid and brief; for others, like the redwood trees, many centuries may elapse. For humans, normal aging extends over many years, and in some cases it exceeds a century. Thus, barring death by accident, war, disease, or inherited life-limiting ailments, each of us has, at birth, the potential for reaching old age. This approach to aging evades the notion of stages and focuses on life-flow, perhaps likening the image of life to a meandering river with both smooth and rough places, divisions and confluences, with all parts contributing to what it becomes before it merges and loses identity in the sea. And the stream is always the stream—the length of flow or the inputs that enrich it do not change that fact. The person is always the person. Experience may contribute to the richness of personality, but within the elder is the youth who is now wiser and more capable because of involvement with the affairs of living. Elders do not lose the basic social and physical needs or the need to be valued as persons. These are fundamental to our humanness.

We are complex creatures, we humans, molded in part by nature and by society, but each uniquely different from the other. Individual experiences coupled with our particular genetic heritage contribute to our distinct one-of-a-kind identity. This concept of aging will surface from time to time in discussions about elders, for according to Nancy A. Newton et al., "There is more diversity among people over sixty-five than any other age group" (1984, p. 231).

This book views elders as those who have entered the last phases of human development. They represent the stream at its fullest flow carrying all the rich and varied experiences of the past into the present. Sometimes they are subdivided into the "young-old" (those sixty-five to seventy-five), and the "old-old" (those over seventy-five). They have left their imprint on every phase of life on earth and have contributed to the extension of the human outreach into space. Theirs are the shoulders upon which younger generations rest, just as these elders stood on the shoulders of their forebears. Like the tidal washes of the ocean, each generation leaves a watermark that can be read by all who care to examine it, depicting the cultural, social, and creative levels reached. What the world is today represents the watermarks of the present generation of elders and constitutes the heritage that the group passes on to those who follow.

To understand the elders of the twentieth century it is important to know who they are, to be aware of where they came from, to understand what they did or failed to do, and to determine how they were affected by the course of both personal and world events. Such an inquiry reveals the characteristics and accomplishments of one of the most remarkable generations in human history. In 1970, Margaret Mead wrote that the eighty-year-olds have "traversed the greatest and most rapid change the world has ever known . . . have crossed more boundaries more successfully and learned to live with more funny kind of things and more strange people they never dreamed of meeting than have the young" (1970, pp. 16–17). Now, some twenty years later, we can say more changes have been compressed into the lifetime of those who are sixty-five years of age and older in the year 1992 than ever before in the history of humankind. Of course, the beginnings and evolution of these innovations can be read in books. What cannot be read is the excitement of being part of and living through the dramatic changes. This can be known and felt only through conversations with the elders. They were there. They can tell us what it was like to be there. As we listen, we gain insight that helps in understanding who the elders are and what they represent.

HOW WE HAVE CHANGED!

The youth of today live in the information age, in a world of immediate communication. Television brings into our living rooms pictures of events occurring in far off places. A 1989 student revolt in China is witnessed by the world, and no matter how the leaders try to camouflage what took place, millions of people have seen for themselves the mustering of troops, that marvelous picture of one young man standing before the advancing tanks, and the brutal quelling of the students' democratic efforts. Contrast that image with those who once listened to news through earphones attached to a crystal-set radio as they moved one wire over a tiny magnet to locate stations and moved another across a coil of wire to amplify and clarify the voices of announcers. Contrast the rapid transoceanic flight of the supersonic Concorde with the slow passage of steamships, or the swift movement from place to place by automobile over paved highways with travel by horse and buggy. How did these changes come about? Ask the elders. It was their generation that initiated and coped with them.

Ask the elders about changes in food habits. They will tell about home canning of fruits and vegetables so that the bounty of the summer could be enjoyed during the winter. They will talk of the transformations of the icebox and the icehouse into the electric refrigerator and freezer, about the preservation of foods by flash-freezing and of the wonder of being able to purchase fresh garden produce throughout the year as the agricultural productivity of one hemisphere where the growing season is in full bloom is transferred to the other hemisphere, which is still gripped by winter. What is now taken for granted, they initiated and lived through.

Think of the international nature of our eating habits. There are few centers in the modern world where Mexican, Japanese, Chinese, European foods, in fresh or frozen form, are not available. In addition, because of the migration of peoples, most large cities have restaurants featuring the cuisine of many nations. Meals need never be monotonous, as they may have been for some elders. Think of the human inventiveness that lies behind the transformation of the same grains and meats into a multitude of different dishes to produce a menu so long that it staggers the imagination! How did this happen? It came out of the lifetime of the elders, who introduced these wonderful exchanges and, for the most part, enjoyed them when they came about.

If you want to engage in an animated dialogue, just ask a group of elders how to "pluck a chicken." Most young people haven't a clue what this phrase means. They think of chicken as something purchased in the poultry section of the supermarket, where it comes plastic-wrapped sans feathers, cleaned and ready for cooking. They have never had to de-feather a dead bird. But many elders have. When I raised the question in one session of mixed ages, a young woman came up and asked in a whisper, "What is a *pin*-feather?" I could have said, "Ask one of the elders," but since I *am* an elder I told her that the pin-feathers were those undeveloped feathers just breaking through the skin of the bird; they remained after the developed feathers were removed. Often they were pulled out with tweezers, but today they are not seen in the birds bought in the markets. The elders have lived through many amazing changes in the handling of food.

The whole pattern of household chores has undergone tremendous changes, too. Electric washing machines and dryers have replaced washboards, tubs, and clotheslines. They had to because World War II forced many women into the factories to replace the men who were in battle zones. Household tasks had to be streamlined, and in so doing freedom from the struggle with time-consuming household tools marked the continuing emancipation of women.

Remember, it was not until after World War I that American women were permitted to vote. That may seem incredible today but the freedom to vote, to work, and to be one's female self was initiated by the elders. Ask them what it was like when they were twenty years of age. Ask about courtship and marriage and how they learned about sex. Learn the history of the dramatic growth and change engendered during this century from those who were part of the change.

Ask about industrial changes. Small mom-and-pop groceries have given way to huge merchandising chains that remain open day and night. Technical enterprises that were once done by hand in small factories are accomplished by multinational corporations using everything from computers to robots. Elders brought these changes into being. It was their creativeness and enterprise that made change take place.

But there is more to the experience of elders than developing and expanding the great societal innovations; there are the personal experiences so unique and so different from those of most modern young people that they can only be heard with fascination and wonder. The elders knew a time when there were vacant lots on most city streets where local youth gathered to play baseball. An entertaining evening could be spent watching magic lantern slides. Then came silent black and white movies, then technicolor, then television. In their day, city families kept chickens and grew vegetables in their back yards. When infectious diseases like scarlet fever or diphtheria struck, homes were quarantined and placed off-limits to everyone in the neighborhood. Elders still harbor the painful memories of the deaths of family members and playmates from these dreadful diseases, most of which are rarely mentioned today. They survived the Great Depression, a time when bright young classmates dropped out of school to work long hours to help support their families. This was a time when shoes wore thin and cardboard or heavy paper covered holes in the soles. This was a time when waste was not condoned and survival required the saving and reuse of what today is treated as disposable, including such mundane things as string, foil, and wrapping paper. Some will remember World War I, when their fathers went to war. All will remember World War II, when young men who had survived the depression were called into military service, when the unemployed became employed as soldiers, when women joined the work force in droves performing tasks that had once been denied to them. All of this seems to have occurred a long time ago, but not for the elders; it is part of their life history. What occurred then has helped to shape our world today—both society and the elders themselves. They have known death and sorrow, divorce and remarriage, widowhood and loneliness, fun and pain, excitement and despair—they are the survivors, and our first concern will be with the ethics of survival.

So elders have lived a long time and have witnessed changes! Big deal! Have they learned anything significant, anything that might contribute to our time? For some there has come an appreciation for the experience and a quiet wisdom born of reflection, and perhaps these concepts are enough to suggest that elders might have something to say to the up-coming generations. On the occasion of his ninety-fifth birthday, Wilbur H. Long, Professor Emeritus of philosophy at the University of Southern California, reflects both in a letter written to a colleague:

> Those of us who were born before or around the turn of the 20th century enjoy, I think, the special favor of Destiny. We have lived in an era of radical change that I suspect is unrepeatable. We came into a world of horse-and-buggy, gas light (even in the street lamps), hot water from the kitchen stove, a four-day trip from Los Angeles to New York, horse-drawn fire engines (and some street cars), luminiferous ether, naive Darwinism (still with us) and Jim Jeffries, but have lived to share a world of nuclear fission, microchips, heart transplants, a new Russia and Orient, DNA and genes, quantum mechanics and relativity, Margaret Thatcher and General Powell.
>
> This contrast of chiaroscuro during the past century evokes in those

of us who have lived through all or most of it a unique sense of history and a vivid awareness of the amazing transformation of things during our lives; whereas the younger folk are more likely to take it all for granted. Moreover, we antiques have shared in those supreme yearnings that man formerly believed to be hopeless, that is, to get to the moon and to fly like a bird, whose fulfillment is likely to turn the triumphs of the future into an anticlimax. And furthermore, whereas we know they will come, our forebears could not even imagine the possibility.

But in spite of this epoch of magic, as Francis Bacon put it, we aged ones who are thoughtful cannot leave the earth and our fellows with satisfaction and hope that are unmitigated. Although on the outside our "progress" is astonishing, we do not see within us all a corresponding advance in serenity, honor, kindness, gratifying existence, or cosmic consciousness. (1991, p. 12f)

How deep is the concern of elders for the world they have developed and for what they have transferred to the future! How bleak and tragic it will be for the future if that delicious savouring of life and the supreme values mentioned by Professor Long should be lost in the race for "progress"!

CONCERNING FACTS AND FIGURES

Demographic studies provide important statistics that enable us to forecast the shape of things to come. There was a time, not so very many years ago, when age sixty-five was considered to be the time to retire. Some elders retired before reaching that age. Some had accumulated what appeared to be enough money to assure a comfortable living for the rest of their lives, augmented by Social Security (to which they had contributed) and by pension plans (to which they and their employers had contributed). Some, compelled to retire at sixty-five, resented this forced alteration of life patterns. Then, changes occurred. Today it is not necessary to retire at this predetermined age; elders well into their eighties are engaged in work for profit because they want to or because they need the income. The change from compulsory retirement has important ethical overtones in that it removed from elders the notion of being "over the hill," no longer contributing to society. It took them out of the category of "unemployable" and provided a choice hitherto denied—to retire or not retire. Furthermore, it removed elders from placement in a statistical box purely on the basis of age, because it confused the data; elders over sixty-five were no longer simply "retirees."

Today more people become elders than ever before in human history. It is a well-advertised fact that patterns of life expectancy at birth have undergone dramatic shifts. A child born in 1900 had a life expectancy of forty-seven years; a newborn today can expect to live well into the late seventies—a more than twenty-five-year increase. However, a person who reached sixty-five years of age in 1900 had a twelve-year life expectancy, while one who reaches the same in 1990 has a fifteen-year life expectancy—an increase of only a few more years. While more people live longer, we have really not been successful in overcoming the factors that terminate the lives of elders (Burnside 1981, pp. 5–7).

In 1900 those sixty-five and older constituted 4.1 percent of the population; in 1970, 10.4 percent; and in 1990, 11.5 percent. By the year 2000 the percentage will rise to 20 percent. This last figure is based on the assumption that fewer people will be inhaling tobacco smoke (directly or indirectly); that there will be a reduction in alcohol consumption; that diet and exercise habits will improve; and that there will be less pollution of air, water, and soil. What is most interesting is that the growth in numbers of persons over seventy-five years of age (sometimes called the old-old group) will increase by 75 percent between 1980 and the end of the century (Burnside 1981, pp. 5–7).

What these figures immediately bring to mind are questions pertaining to income (with particular reference to Social Security in the United States) and health, most particularly in the United States which is one of the two first world countries that has failed to develop a national health insurance program (the other country being South Africa). All other first world countries protect their citizens with national health coverage. At this point, the ethical issue of survival comes into focus.

The ethical question that confronts us is just what, if anything, does society owe these remarkable elders who have survived into the last decade of the twentieth century? This question will be discussed later.

It is important to acknowledge that aging does not signify changes within the person. Most changes are external and are forced upon elders by a society that is out of touch with the reality of age (see chapter 4 on "Agism"). Alex Comfort put it this way:

> Aging has no effect upon you as a person. When you are "old" you will feel no different and be no different from what you are now or were when you were young, except that more experiences will have happened. In age your appearance will change, however, and you may encounter more physical problems. When you do, these will affect you

only as physical problems affect a person of any age. An "aged" person is simply a person who has been there longer than a young person. (p. 28)

Elders have the same basic needs for food, clothing, security, health, respect, and meaning in their lives as the young. When these are denied, thwarted, or ignored, and when an elder's unique life story or his/her role in the collective history of this remarkable generation is ignored or dismissed as irrelevant, then the question of ethical treatment of elders is raised.

REFERENCES

Burnside, Irene M., ed. 1981. *Nursing and the Aged.* New York: McGraw-Hill.

Comfort, Alex. 1976. *A Good Age.* New York: Crown Publishers, Inc.

Lamont, Corliss. 1981. *Yes to Life: Memories of Corliss Lamont.* New York: Horizon Press.

Long, Wilbur H. 1991. "Letter" in *Retired Faculty Association Newsletter,* University of Southern California, March-April, pp. 12f.

Mead, Margaret. 1970. "The Cultural Shaping of the Ethical Situation," in Kenneth Vaux, ed., *Who Shall Live?* Philadelphia, Fortress Press, pp. 4–23.

Newton, Nancy A., Lawrence W. Lazarus, and Jack Weinberg. 1984. "Aging: Biosocial Perspectives," in Daniel Offer and Melvin Sabshin, *Normality and the Life Cycle.* New York: Basic Books, Publishers.

3

The Elders as Citizens: Human Rights

"And crown thy good, with brotherhood,
From sea to shining sea."

—Katherine Lee Bates, "America the Beautiful," 1895

Free nations have produced slogans that epitomize the rights, privileges, and dreams of the citizenry. In France, the words, "Liberty, Equality, and Fraternity" symbolize a national ethos. In the United States of America, a government of the people, by the people, and for the people is designed to protect rights to "life, liberty, and the pursuit of happiness." The Canadian Constitution provides for freedom of conscience, religion, thought, belief, opinion, expression, and association. It states further that everyone has the right to "life, liberty, and security" (Boyajian, p. 27). The list could be expanded. Each statement pertains to a life ethic, to a survival ethic recognizing that the healthy human psyche requires something beyond bare existence. For example, the notion of a "right to life" reflects basic survival needs and implies the right to resources for adequate food, clothing, shelter, and safety. Without these, democratic existence would be impossible and life would surely be reduced to the survival of the fittest with the strongest in control.

The constitutional guarantee of freedom implies that each individual, regardless of age, social status, wealth, religion, ethnicity or sexual identity should have the opportunity to become what he or she wants to be and, under ordinary circumstances, is at liberty to pursue any chosen life course. Individuals are free to make choices regarding personal well-being, insofar as those choices do not inhibit or infringe on the rights and freedoms of others. They are free to express points of view, to follow their beliefs, to support causes they believe in, to meet with others who share similar views, and to organize support for their concepts. The freedom to be recognizes that self-fulfillment and self-actualization are individual needs of the psyche that go beyond the physical and will vary from person to person.

The concept of fraternity acknowledges the human need for companionship. It recognizes that to express our full humanity we have a need to belong. By implication there is an awareness of the social and psychological dangers of isolation and loneliness, both of which will be discussed later.

These declarations of human rights constitute basic value statements. When they are applied to the lives of elders, their implementation raises ethical issues. Whenever freedoms are curtailed or frustrated, the human psyche is damaged, the personality withers, and the individual cannot live up to his or her highest potential. How can such basic psychological, social, and civil rights, and the needs of elders be protected and articulated?

THE DREAM AND THE REALITY

Social policies, the organizing principles that provide guides to actions affecting citizens as individuals or groups, reflect governmental desires to correct inequities, to improve the conditions of the disadvantaged, and provide assistance to the weaker or less powerful (Morris 1979, p. 1). Sometimes these policies emerge after a situation that has been developing over a long period of time reaches crisis proportions. At other times, emerging societal patterns give forewarning of problems to be met and planned for before they become formidable. Social concerns relating to the well-being of the elderly fall into this latter category.

Demographic studies chart the tremendous increase in numbers of elderly persons who will confront local, national, and world policy makers in the twenty-first century. One hundred years ago, only 2 percent of Americans were over the age of sixty-five. By the turn of the century, this figure had increased to 4 percent. Today more than 11 percent of the population is over sixty-five and there is a net gain of more than one thousand entering the ranks of these elders every day. By the year 2000, it is expected that more than 20 percent of the population will be seventy-five years of age or older (Berkow 1987, p. 2390).

Emerging social problems demand immediate solutions even as they foreshadow the complexity and deepening of these issues in the future. The problems include adequate food, shelter, clothing, security, and health care; provision for the opportunity for a meaningful existence with the right of the competent elder to choose for the self; and the provision of durable power of attorney, particularly in the area of health care, should the elder become incompetent. For the very wealthy, these needs can be met on an individual or family basis; for the poor or less wealthy, governmental assistance will be necessary.

The millions of homeless or street people, ranging in age from the very young to the very old, testify to a social disregard of basic human needs for food, clothing, and lodging. When the number of reported accounts of elder abuse continue to rise, when elders are physically, psychologically, financially, and spiritually damaged—either through direct action or through neglect—a social statement is being made.

In the 1960s, social awareness of child abuse prompted the passing of laws to protect the children and the establishment of places of refuge for abused youngsters. In the 1970s, the evidence of widespread spouse abuse led to the development of laws and havens of security for abused women and their children. In the 1980s, case after case of reported elder abuse made us aware that the elderly may be listed among the vulnerable and poorly protected members of society. Since then some regulations seeking to protect elders have been developed.

The effects of elder abuse are like those experienced by defenseless children and spouses and are characterized by diminished feelings of self-worth. As the quality of life fades, existence becomes burdensome. Whatever contributions abused elders may have made to society throughout their long lives are negated and rendered meaningless; elders shrink socially, spiritually, and psychologically. Most elder abuse is engendered within families but there are enough reports from nursing homes and retirement communities to raise concern.

Some abuse of elders occurs in families where abrasive and abusive practices have a long history and, indeed, may have been initiated by the elders themselves when they were younger and in control of the family. Consequently some elder abuse takes the form of revenge. A folk-rhyme puts it this way:

> When I was a laddie, I lived with my granny,
> And many a hiding, my granny did give me.
> Now I'm a man, and I live with my granny,
> I do to my granny what she did to me.

In other cases, violence is accepted as a standard familial way to solve problems, including those associated with elders. Sometimes a change in relationships with elders occurs during periods of financial, familial, or social stress. Unemployment by the breadwinners makes the elder's retirement money important to the family as a whole; an elder may be deprived of needed medications and proper foods as his/her limited income goes to support others. Alcohol and drug abuse by family members lowers inhibitory barriers, with elders becoming targets of drunken or drug-induced anger. If responsibility for elder care is shifted to grandchildren, the elder becomes a bothersome nuisance who interrupts the young peoples' schedules. In such cases, the frail or dependent elder may be neglected and mistreated.

THE DEPENDENT ELDER

Life isn't easy for anyone when an elder becomes dependent, frail, and needy. If the ailing person were a child, attention would be willingly given in the anticipation of recovery. With weak and ailing elders, however, the health trajectory is toward death. Now, the elder person who, in the mind of his or her children, had always appeared as a capable and self-contained adult, becomes as helpless as a child. The role of children parenting their parents—caring for them, advising them, looking after them as if they were infants—becomes a social anomaly in which normal patterns are turned upside down. One man reported the stress he and his family experienced as they cared for his two weak and ailing parents in their home for more than two years. While his wife and children were responsible during the day, he tried to assume care during evenings and at night, often being deprived of sleep as he responded to his parents' needs for care and attention. He acted out of love for his parents and they lived at his home because he could not afford the high cost of nursing home or hospital care. They died nine months apart, but for twenty-six months his life and the life of his family was locked in to the care of these two elderly persons.

Not every family is emotionally equipped to deal with live-in elders. A married woman, responsible for two teenaged children and a husband in the initial stages of what has been diagnosed as probable terminal cancer, watches with concern as her aging parents suffer one ailment after another. Should they become incapacitated or, should one of them die, she would be the person responsible for their care or for nurturing the survivor. Her present responsibilities are overwhelming. Her parents have always been demanding people. She anticipates the future with fear and uncertainty.

An eighty-four-year-old woman has been informed by her niece that her eighty-two-year-old sister, the niece's mother, is incapable of taking care of herself and that it is her responsibility as the sister to look after the ailing woman. Family loyalty and feelings of duty conflict with the knowledge of her inability to provide the care necessary for her sister's well-being. The niece refuses to take her mother into her home because she has enough responsibilities with her husband and her children.

Often when familial care is undertaken the stress on the supporting family is almost unbearable. A twenty-eight-year-old woman, completing her doctorate degree, is responsible not only for her mother, who is dying of smoking-induced cancer, but also a father who has had a colostomy and is trying to cope with his own discomfort and the trauma of his hospitalized, dying wife. The family is not poor and household help is available. But the physical and emotional drain of hospital visits; academic pressures; and a demanding, chronically ill father bring on weight loss and the need for stabilizing medications in the daughter. Her intentions are good, she is loyal and loving, but, as she puts it, the demands are "too much."

An eighty-five-year-old woman has Alzheimer's disease and has decayed mentally and physically to the point where she lies in a hospital bed comatose and unaware of the world, which she had long since forgotten. Her devoted eighty-seven-year-old husband visits each day spending hours at her bedside, sometimes talking softly, though long before her hospitalization she had ceased to recognize him. He is angry and upset that his children and grandchildren do not want to visit the frail old woman.

Respite care can be important. Where the caregiving family is isolated from other relatives who might, on a one-day-per-week basis, take over care, only hired professionals, paid out of personal savings or government funds, or provided by church groups, can rescue the overburdened family. Without such help the potential for stress-related abuse becomes a real possibility—even in the most loving of families.

WHO CARES?

The ethics of survival are complex. What is the duty of children to their parents? What ethical choices for health care are provided and how does one choose? Does society owe elders anything? Can it be assumed that the comatose woman with Alzheimer's has outlived her usefulness and that her life has no meaning? Should she be given a lethal injection and permitted to die? Who would or could make such a decision? What do the great democratic themes of life, liberty, freedom, fraternity, and the search for happiness mean when one becomes old and feeble? Do such slogans have any meaning for elders?

The degree to which the nation provides an opportunity for the individual to achieve, acquire, or fulfill the ideal of the national ethic as expressed in formal declarations testifies to the validity of the proclamation. The extent to which citizens (in this case, elders) are prevented, hindered, or limited in maximizing their opportunities to fulfill the dream of life, liberty, and the pursuit of happiness, characterizes the failure of the national ethic. The growing number of elders who are and have been frustrated in their efforts to live a full life, a decent life, a secure life, raises serious questions about the meaning of slogans that give lip service to commitment to the quality of human existence.

If the present failures were not discouraging enough, awareness of the swelling ranks of elders that will occur in the near future—and whose numbers will only serve to increase the ranks of unfulfilled lives—can only engender feelings of helplessness and hopelessness for many fine, decent human beings in the years ahead. In the United States, one of the richest and most powerful nations on earth, the failure to meet elder needs to exist on a level free of fear and of poverty, with adequate health care and security from abuse, constitutes a national tragedy and a moral disgrace.

REFERENCES

Berkow, Robert. 1987. *The Merck Manual.* New Jersey: Merck and Co. Inc.

Morris, Robert. 1979. *Social Policy of the American Welfare State.* New York: Harper and Row.

4

Geroethics and Agism

"Attitudes toward old age vary as widely as definitions of it. American society, as well as most modernized societies, is generally negative toward it. We glorify youth and despise old age. We associate old age with loss of usefulness, decrepitude, illness, senility, poverty, loss of sexuality, sterility, and death. As a result, people take great pains to preserve a youthful appearance and conceal or understate their actual chronological age."

—Donald O. Cowgill, *Aging Around the World,* p. 8

THE ELDER AS A "GROUPIE"

The term "groupie" is generally applied to teenage devotees of some rock star or those who cluster around some cult leader. I suppose that in a sense, we are all, by nature, "groupies." From our beginning, we are born into, live with, and think in terms of, groups. Most of us come into the world as a member of a family that may be small and isolated or large and embracing depending upon whether it is nuclear or extended. We immediately inherit our race, our citizenship, our nationality, our community (deep south, east or west coast, and so forth), and our culture. As we mature we become members of school and religious clubs, Boy or Girl Scouts, teams, musical assemblages, art circles, political parties, and associations related to the way in which we earn our living. In other words, throughout our lives, we become members of one group or another.

Groups may provide a basis for self-identification. Depending on their status, they contribute to feelings of self-worth. The teenaged groupie has an identification as a follower or supporter of some star or idol. On a more mature level, when social issues surface, the influence of a community of people may be necessary to have a particular point of view recognized. Each group has its special identity that distinguishes it from others, and each has within it the potential for developing arguments supporting discrimination against outsiders.

In other words, from birth we are taught to think in terms of group relationships. We are comfortable within our own group. But we may feel ill at ease among those who use a different language, embrace different slogans, or represent different interests. We learn to evaluate these "others" in terms of broad generalities or stereotypes, some of which may be untrue and even denigrating.

When tensions arise—be they local, national, or international—prejudicial and stereotypical thinking surfaces so that an identified body of people may be characterized in ways that devalue and dehumanize. "They" are responsible for the decline in values. "They" are responsible for our financial woes. "They" are sucking the lifeblood from society or are tax burdens or are in one way or another categorized as problems. Thus, while there are strengthening merits in group thinking, there are also dangerous, divisive, and destructive potentials.

Elders compose an identifiable group based solely on age. There may be subdivisions according to health or race or religion or place of residence, but, in general, elders are grouped together as those over the age of sixty-five. In this sense elders become "groupies."

AGISM

Agism (a term coined by Robert N. Butler in 1967) is the negative attitudinal response toward elders that demeans and dehumanizes them. Agism classifies elders as a group. It thrives on stereotypes expressed in language, labels, gestures, humor, practices, policies and even advocacy. It is found in the home, the school, the media, the marketplace, and in hospitals, nursing homes, and governmental circles. Its practitioners represent children and youth (taught by adults), the middle-aged, and even some elders themselves, any one of whom may be illiterate or well-educated, a blue-collar or white-collar worker, therapists, professionals, or legislators, and of any race or creed or political affiliation. The effects of agism are toxic for the individual in particular, for elders in general, and for society as a whole inasmuch as agism represents a bigotry that separates elders from society's protective norms rendering them vulnerable and, in some instances, helpless. Agism is unethical.

STEREOTYPES

Agism, as a form of stereotypical thinking, avoids recognition of individual features or attributes. Elders are depicted as physically (and often mentally) feeble or retarded, as unattractive, as those who slow progress, and as parasites living on public welfare. When surveys regarding images of or attitudes toward aging are taken, negative aspects of becoming old always outweigh positive ones. When members of a group are asked to visualize old age, the images reported include wrinkles, bent bodies, feebleness, hearing loss, toothlessness, gnarled and stiffened hands, a shuffling gate, loneliness, boredom, poverty, white hair, failing eyesight, loss of memory, and senility.

Advertisers of beauty aids enhance this negative image of elders as they encourage sales by threatening their readers or listeners with the ravages of age that can only be bypassed by using their particular products. We are warned to beware of acquiring wrinkles, age spots, graying hair, and so on. The message is clear: aging is a negative process and growing old is the equivalent of becoming ugly and undesirable. Such promotional advertising not only underscores the emphasis on youth culture but affects the ways in which people think about aging in general and about their own aging in particular.

No one of us is completely immune to the advertising that bombards us visually and audibly every day. No one wants to be perceived as "ugly." Product manufacturers and their advertising agents tap into these fears. They have a ready-made, lucrative market among those elderly who buy into the projected negative images. Of course, advertising promises are never completely fulfilled. Age spots may fade, but they remain. Gray hair may be transformed into any color, but it is still there. Wrinkles really do not disappear—they may be hidden for a short time, but they are still present and will continue increasing in number. What the public in general and elders in particular need to accept and recognize is the beauty present in the aged. Each age group has its own special beauty. Elder beauty is not that of the middle-aged, the teenager, or the infant. It has its own comeliness and proportions. Some elders are proud of their gray hair and wrinkled countenances, which are testimonials to their journey through life. It is the sort of beauty we recognize in gnarled oak trees, giant redwoods, and other natural statements of aging.

At the same time, there is nothing to be condemned in the efforts of elders to look their best. If that effort involves dyeing hair, the use of creams and other so-called beauty-aids, there is nothing to criticize. Many simply continue patterns enjoyed throughout their lifetimes. What is unethical is to suggest that not trying to change one's aging appearance, or not using the advertised product, is some kind of demotion to ugliness. Aging, wrinkled faces, gray hair, and hands marked with brown spots have their own special beauty.

The language of agism, which is extensive and pervasive, characterizes ways of thinking about elders. Some of the terms are: "relic of the past" or "old relic," "out-of-date," "not-with-it," "old fossil," "obsolete," "over-the-hill," "old fogey," "old codger," "old crock," "crotchety," "decrepit," "doddering," "graybeard," "senile," "outmoded," "little old lady/man," "wizened," "wrinkled," "superannuated," "archaic," "second childhood," "dotage," "past the prime," "having one foot in the grave," "antiquated," and on and on. One need only pause and more terms come to mind "withered," "toothless," "old biddy"—the list seems endless. Each label can be used to negate the significance of an elder.

Societal attitudes are reflected in the ways in which we approach certain ages. There is something exciting about an eighteenth or twenty-first birthday. Both are associated with expanded privileges. But when these same persons become twenty-nine and approach their thirtieth birthday, they express uncertainty—feelings we can perhaps associate with youths warning in the 1960s not to trust anyone over thirty. Then, when these people are thirty-nine, the fortieth birthday can become a symbol of final decay, because somehow we have associated age forty with a middle point and with the beginning of decline. In actuality, most of these anxious adults discover that no drastic changes have occurred in the transitions. Some will pretend to remain 29 or 39 for many years, thereby testifying to their fear and denial of aging. Such toxic attitudes do not nourish the quality of life and living; in fact, they can rob existence of the healthy, life-fulfilling attitudes and experiences associated with aging.

Even among gerontologists, where such general projections are denied, some demographers have produced age caste systems—one would label elders as "young-old," old, and "old-old," which once again tends to encourage treating individuals according to age groups rather than as individuals. Of course, age classifications can have importance for projecting population changes, but if gerontologists insist on utilizing such distributions, then the categories need to be expanded. For example, a specific individual might be identified as follows: "m-y/o-pl-el0-ph-nsf" (male, young-old, poverty level, education 10 years, poor health, nonsupportive family) to distinguish the person from "f-y/o-mi-e12-gh-sf" (female, young-old, middle income, education twelve years, good health, supportive family). The only figure in common is the age bracket, everything else differs. Even with this breakdown, one needs definitions of what is meant by terms like "poor health" and "poverty level." The more we utilize stereotypes the more we deny and ignore the person and individual differences.

Some labels may or may not be offensive. A person may be a Canadian or an American or a Mexican, and depending on the current local attitude toward any specific nationality, the label is acceptable and convenient. But one need only recall the rather silly and demeaning Polish "jokes" that used to circulate or the cruel Hollywood cartoon portrayals of Orientals to recognize the ways in which a dominant society may humiliate its minorities.

WHY STEREOTYPES?

Why do we engage in destructive stereotypes? Negative labels reflect insecurity and are, perhaps, expressions of fear. They enable one group to assert power or superiority by demeaning another. The need to make demeaning assertions reflects the insecurity of the labeler.

Agist remarks represent a denial growing out of fear of aging. If one can distance oneself from aging by mocking or denigrating elders, the negative reaction serves as a protective barrier against aging: after all, most ego-centered persons do not mock or demean themselves. Elders are made to represent that which is other, rather than that which one will become. Once the language is accepted, elders are automatically pigeonholed no matter whether or not they fit. For example, thanks to progress in modern living, health standards, and medical research, many humans live longer than ever before and thus the "old-old" group is growing rapidly. But what does the label suggest? Just what is "old-old" beyond being someone eighty-five or older?

What if the eighty-six-year-old's blood pressure is 125/76 and the person has low cholesterol, is trim, moderately athletic, manages an office or a business, and is happy and satisfied with life and living? What does "old-old" convey? Further, how does the general stereotype fit? Do gray hairs and wrinkles contribute to the labelling? Stereotypes have destructive potential, whether held by the public at large or by researchers in the field of aging. They tend to force noncompliant individuals into wasted efforts to prove they do not fit the mold or perhaps into simply giving up and accepting the image and conforming to it. Just think of those who are old-old. How does the eighty-six-year-old described above fit the mental image of "old-old"? Who would hire or even bother interviewing this person after reading the dossier that described a vibrant, creative, and self-possessed person who is nonetheless categorized as "old-old"? Who would grant such an individual any social responsibility? It is demographically necessary to recognize aging trajectories, but it is important to be aware of the damage to the ego, to feelings of self-esteem, and to the way in which elders are perceived and treated when stereotyped. Cataloguing does not explain who or what the person is; it only classifies the individual as a member of an age group. When the group is deemed to have certain general characteristics, individuals are labeled willy-nilly.

AGISM IN CORPORATE AMERICA

Corporate America practices agism. Dianne Klein reported case after case in which she noted "Gray hair can wash years of success down the drain" (1990). Vince Boyle had been a vice president for human resources:

> At 56 years old, Vince Boyle was too old, a virtual relic in the leaner, meaner world of corporate America. His company, an international firm in Newport Beach, preferred to call his departure part of a reorganization.
> "I was the only one who had gray hair and some of them were older than me, Boyle says. "This was a joke in our company. Then you see them on the street, after we were all let go, and they all look like me. They were dyeing their hair." (Klein 1990)

What do elders do when they are "relieved" of their positions? They send out résumés and find they are "over qualified"—a polite form of rejection. They sell their homes, and maybe they work in supermarkets at $5.75 an hour, supervised by department managers who are less than half their age and with less than half their experience and know-how. These unemployed and unemployable elders are, according to one, "part of a throwaway society. They should use us for Earth Day, recycle us" (Klein 1990). Despite rejection and feelings of uselessness, some elders can still keep their sense of humor!

THE PATRONIZED ELDER

Elder humor, which is often debasing, is not new. For centuries bawdy tales have poked fun at impotence or described aging bodies in deprecating ways. In folk humor, elders are the gullible ones. Elder males who marry younger women are cuckolded while elder females are used. Elders who try to pass themselves off as younger than they are become subjects of crude mockery.

In numerous television sit-coms, elders shuffle (just as stereotyped Afro-Americans did in early movies), are shrill voiced or so hard of hearing that they must be shouted at, or are semi-senile. In commercials, older adults are often funny little old ladies who demand "Where's the beef?" or eat food with strange gestures. In comic strips, they are grumpy school bus drivers; possessive, controlling Mommas; or boring, long-winded, and preachy women, like Mary Worth. Such images do not enhance; instead, they demean and cater to the stereotypes. Of course some elder humor and some advertisements depict normal individuals, but so long as the portrayal of elders is distorted, older persons will continue to be demeaned.

If this were not enough, elders are often patronized. Elder women lose their identity and become "dearie" or "honey," in settings ranging from the marketplace to hospitals and nursing homes. They are treated like children or as feeble incompetents. Older women seem to be stereotyped more often than men. In case after case, older women have reported that when their spouse is hospitalized and they seek out information concerning his illness (e.g., the prognostications and so forth), they are either patronized and treated as mental incompetents, or they are labelled hysterical, perhaps on the assumption that women are, by nature, emotionally unstable (another nonsensical stereotype). Men get the "pops" treatment by a wide range of people, from garage mechanics to waitresses. When they lodge protests against such harassment many older men are labeled as "acting up-tight" and are informed that the person "didn't mean anything by the term." The implication is that the elder is overreacting and should simply relax and be "normal" or accepting.

Tokenism, by which elders are granted some small voice in the management of their lives or in the administration of institutions where they are compelled to reside, diminishes feelings of worth and insults the ability of many older people to assume responsibility by implying a lack of rational or ethical perspective. Retirement communities can benefit from resident input. Nursing homes that make only token provision for residents to participate in management and social issues affecting their lives reduce the status of elders to incompetent objects of care and, in so doing, increase feelings of helplessness.

Even the segregation of elders in villages and housing units for those "fifty-five and over" can represent a form of agism. But older people may choose such segregated living for a variety of reasons. Some do not want children around. They have raised their families, and thoughts of babies crying in the night, the often shrill noise of children at play, or of teen music, are simply unacceptable. They prefer to be separated. Others move into special low-cost housing for economic reasons, not simply to get away from other age groups. They do not necessarily believe that elders prefer their own company.

In a conference setting, one director of low-cost housing for elders told of a one-week visit by her daughter and grandchild. A few resident elders suggested that the visiting daughter and child should not be allowed to stay in the director's apartment. On the other hand, others were drawn to the three-year-old grand-daughter, an attractive, gregarious child, who simply accepted all elders as additional grandparents. After the daughter and child left, the residents talked about the visit for weeks. It would be stereotypical to suggest that all living units should accommodate different age groups. On the other hand, it is equally stereotypical to suggest that most elders prefer to associate only with their own age group.

Any portrayal or treatment that diminishes the image or status or feelings of self-worth of an elder (or of anyone else) is unethical and toxic.

CHANGING ATTITUDES

Can anything be done to raise this level of geroethical thinking? Of course. Like any other bigotry, agism is a learned response, and what has been learned can be unlearned. No society will be completely homogeneous, but every society can learn tolerance, understanding, and harmonious and peaceful ways to come to grips with differences.

Gordon W. Allport (1958), in his study of prejudice, noted that unless the equilibrium of a system is upset, there is a tendency to deny that any problem exists. "Peopl are so accustomed to the prevailing system of caste and discrimination that they think it is eternally fixed and entirely satisfactory to all concerned" (p. 464). He notes that "even in communities seething with prejudice" there is a denial that prejudice exists (p. 465). How can the situation be changed?

The countering of agism must have several approaches. The first is to attack blatant examples through the press; through publicized meetings; letters of protest to congressmen and senators; and by appeal to national standards of democracy, decency, and respect. Simultaneously, education about the facts needs to be clearly offered. For example, at the present moment, complaints about Social Security payments to elders continue to surface. Elders need to help complainers understand that they (the elders) and their employers contributed to that fund to make it what it is. They need to point out that the Social Security fund is a rich depository and that there are government officials who are trying to tap into it for purposes other than that for which it was established. In other words, complaints built on rumors need to be countered by fact. Allport (1958, p. 470) found "three benign effects" resulting from the "outpouring of information":

(a) It sustains the confidence of minorities to see an effort being made to counter prejudice with truth.

(b) It encourages and reinforces tolerant people by augmenting their attitudes with knowledge.

(c) It tends to undermine the rationalization of bigots.

Elders have many interests and belong to many religious, social, cultural, environmental, and political organizations. Their very presence in and support of these groups testifies to who they are and what they stand for. Through these associations elders can make their presence felt and their voices heard. When agism raises its ugly head, members of the groups in which elders are active can counter agist stereotypes on the basis of what they know from their experiences with elders.

Older adults are at present in a unique position. Many in Western society have been raised with a commandment to "honor fathers and mothers" so that mistreatment and maltreatment of elders carries some degree of social or religious opprobrium. This, however, is not enough to occasion change, for religious rules have always carried the potential of being ignored.

What is more significant is that the growing number of elders is beginning to provide social clout. Elder voices and responses can be heard and felt in the marketplace and the ballot box. When steps to public buildings are too steep and too numerous, the complaints of elders have resulted in the construction of gently sloping ramps that accommodate wheelchairs and provide a gradual approach to entrances. Elders have even been responsible for prodding public auditoriums to improve their sound systems.

Public restrooms in shopping malls are often located in almost inaccessible locations and may lack such important accessories as grab bars or wheelchair accessibility. Elder requests have resulted in changes that benefited the handicapped as well as older persons. Of course, there is a danger here of a boomerang effect: reaction against elder power can engender the agism stereotype. Elders can be (and have been) labeled negatively and seen as social leeches, nuisances demanding and draining social resources and costing more than they contribute.

Individuals can become involved in reeducation and experimentation in "unlearning"; sometimes the experience can be fun. Let me illustrate by citing a personal experience. Remember the Polish jokes mentioned above? One acquaintance, a Presbyterian minister, had a collection of these and each time he told one, I was irritated. What could I do? I devised the following scheme. Each time this clergyman told a Polish joke, I would comment, "Oh, that's not the way I heard it." I would then retell the story substituting a Presbyterian minister for the Pole. He did not like what he heard. He stopped telling the jokes, at least in my presence, and I rather enjoyed my role as an irritating reeducator.

Sometimes an educational setting can present a challenge. Several years ago, when I was an adjunct professor at the College of Art and Design in Pasadena, California, I asked my class of wonderfully creative students to come back in one week with current images of aging. They brought in montages of collapsing buildings, photos of elders shuffling along the street or standing in the marketplace bewildered and looking lost and so on. They were in touch with society and found these attitudes current. Their next assignment was to come back in one week with ideas that would change stereotypical thinking about elders. The results were striking. Photography majors produced pictures of vibrant, beautiful, wrinkled, gray-haired elders that radiated *joie de vivre* and pictured them doing everything from throwing frisbees to necking in the park. Sketch artists reached out to educate by producing children's coloring books with pictures of active, involved elders who had time to relate to children. Some drew cartoons. In one, an elderly couple were pictured sitting in bed, toasting one another with champagne glasses. The caption read: "It may take a little longer, but its just as good." What a wonderful counter to the image of sexless elders! Inasmuch as these young people would become the media producers of the future, it was important that they recognize the positive elements in the lives of many older persons—a dimension that can readily be lost sight of or ignored through stereotyping.

AGING, AGISM, AND THE REAL THING

It would be folly to ignore the realities of aging. Some elders are feeble, some are crotchety, some have developed asocial stances, some are senile. Indeed, we have a literary heritage that expresses the undesirable aspects of growing old. During the twenty-fifth century B.C.E., Ptah-hotep, the wise old Egyptian vizier wrote:

> Old age has arrived. Elderliness is here. Feebleness has come. Dotage is at hand. Each day the heart (mind) responds drowsily, eyes are weak, ears are deaf, strength is dissipated by weariness. The mouth is silent and cannot speak; the heart (mind) is forgetful and cannot recall yesterday. Bones ache all over, good has become evil. The nose is stuffed up and cannot breathe and taste is gone. What old age does to men is evil in every respect. (Larue 1985)

In another context, Qoheleth, the teacher, who probably lived in the third or fourth century B.C.E., advised his students:

> Remember your grave, while you are young,
> When troublous day are still far off,
> Nor have the years come when you will say
> "I find no pleasure in them";
> Before the sunshine becomes dimmed,
> The light from moon and stars fails
> And the clouds come with rain.
> When that day does comes, house supports (legs) tremble
> and even strong men are bent over.
> The grinders (teeth) cease because they are few
> And those that peer out from windows (eyes) are clouded
> And the doors to the street (ears) are closed
> And the sounds from the mill are hushed,
> Even the song of the bird is silenced
> As are all the sounds of singing daughters.
> Then men are terrified of heights
> Or of whatever may lie in the road,
> Then the white almond tree blossoms (hair)
> Even a grasshopper is a burden.
> Sexual desire fails
> For man is going to his eternal home.
> Mourners wait in the streets
> For the silver cord to be cut, the golden bowl smashed,

The pitcher shattered at the fountain,
The wheel broken at the cistern.
Then (human) dust returns to the earth from whence it came
And the life-breath will return to God who gave it.
(Eccles. 12:1-7)

Playwrights, poets, novelists, philosophers, and psychologists have written of the decline in vigor and health that can come with aging, but these need not become stereotypes unless we let them. It is true that many do not look forward with relish to becoming old, but the ways in which we age vary. Not all fit the ancient images. Unless we move beyond agism, the negative stereotypes will prevail.

Elders would be foolish to deny that some limitations come with aging, and some have recognized these in positive, delightful ways, often with gentle humor. For example someone has written:

My face in the mirror isn't wrinkled or drawn,
My furniture is dusted, the cobwebs are gone.
My garden is lovely; so is my lawn.
Don't think I'll ever put my glasses back on!
(anon.)

Someone else wrote:

Always remember that old folks are worth a fortune, with silver in their hair, gold in their teeth, stones in their kidneys, lead in their feet, and gas in their stomachs.
(Sophia S. Rehman)

THE DANGERS OF AGISM

As with any form of stereotypical thinking, agism bristles with potential dangers. As the elderly population swells to numbers unprecedented in history, and as health and welfare costs mount, attitudes toward elders can change, becoming bitter, destructive, and reactive. Under such circumstances, agism provides a potential for the development of negative and dehumanizing social myths concerning the elderly, just as stereotypes have developed such myths in the past (Milgrim, 1974, pp. 8ff). Social myths assume authority in and of themselves and, consequently, public conformity and obedience to the implications of a negative myth can result in harm to the stereotyped group, in this case, the elders. Because agism tends to devalue the persons as individuals, they become absorbed in the age classification. Devaluation opens the door to insensitivity and provides a basis for ignoring individual needs and social rights. Subjective feelings, which under ordinary circumstances might temper prejudicial responses, tend to become submerged in loyalty to popular concepts, and a group, such as elders, can become the target of public persecution. In times of austerity (especially financial austerity), scapegoating seeks to target groups, particularly those that appear to take from the system without giving in return. Welfare recipients are often singled out for attack. In the future, the swollen numbers of elders, whose health and long-term care needs may place exceptional strains on national budgets, may become scapegoats. In such a setting, past contributions will be set aside, ignored, or forgotten as present costs become the basis for discrimination.

These are harsh warnings, but human history is riddled with vivid examples. There are, moreover, enough bigoted groups in society to serve as harbingers of what attitudes could develop even in the most sensitive and democratic environments. Throughout this book, I will suggest patterns that could forestall overreaction against elders. The first is a warning concerning the potential dangers in stereotyping. The second is awareness of the language of agism. The third is a sensitivity to the harm done by agist thinking, speaking, and acting. Finally, there is the responsibility to react to agism by seeking to eliminate its destructive influence through protest and through raising social consciousness of its presence and toxicity.

REFERENCES

Allport, Gordon W. 1958. *The Nature of Prejudice,* Garden City, N.Y.: Doubleday & Company, Inc. (reprint of 1954 edition).

Braun-Kessler, Julia. 1980. *Getting Even With Getting Old.* New York: Nelson-Hall.

Bulter, Robert N. 1969. "Agism: Another Form of Bigotry," *The Gerontologist* 9, pp. 243–46.

Cole, Thomas R., and Sally A. Gadow. 1986. *What Does It Mean to Grow Old?* Durham, N.C.: Duke University Press.

Cowgill, Donald O. 1986. *Aging Around the World.* Belmont, Calif.: Wadsworth Publishing Company.

Dowd, James J. 1980. *Stratification Among the Aged.* Monterey, Calif.: Brooks/Cole Publishing Co.

Jones, Rochell. 1977. *The Other Generation: The New Power of Older People.* Englewood Cliffs, N.J.: Prentice-Hall.

Klein, Dianne. 1990. "Gray Hair Can Wash Years of Success Down the Drain," *The Los Angeles Times* (Orange County Edition), April 11.

Larue, Gerald A. 1985. "Historical Perspectives on the Role of the Elderly" in Gari Lesnoff-Caravaglia, ed., *Values, Ethics and Aging.* New York: Human Sciences Press, pp. 41-61.

Milgrim, Stanley. 1974. *Obedience to Authority.* New York: Harper and Row.

Nuessel, Frank H., Jr. 1982. "The Language of Ageism," *The Gerontologist* 23, no. 3, pp. 273-75.

Rehman, Sophia S., ed. 1991. *Retired Faculty Association Newsletter,* University of Southern California, March-April, p. 13.

Schonfield, David. 1982. "Who Is Stereotyping Whom and Why?" *The Gerontologist* 22, no. 3, pp. 267-72.

5

The Ethics of Survival

"When you've had a long life and you're ripe, then it's time to go." Massachusets gubernatorial candidate John Silber, sixty-three, on why he supports the rationing of health benefits for the elderly.

—*Newsweek* (July 30, 1990), p. 13

The ethical quality of a nation may be judged in part by the way in which the helpless, the handicapped, and the aged are treated. With notable exceptions (e.g., Rumania) most countries seek ways to protect infants and children. These little ones are important for they will provide the national strength, the work force, the productivity, and the prosperity of the future. The well-being of healthy adults is also a prime concern for they are the producers of national wealth. However, there may be those who by virtue of physical or mental handicaps, or by becoming old, do not command the same protection and care as infants, the young people, and the middle-aged. Care for such persons may require the expenditure of more money than they can earn. At this point the issue of survival ethics becomes paramount.

THE PRINCIPLE OF SURVIVAL

Every living thing adapts to its environment as part of the effort to survive. For example, the late Professor Yigael Yadin told me of his excavation of the ancient fortress of Masada, Israel, in the 1960s. The landscape of that barren, arid outcropping looms over the Dead Sea. Then came an unexpected rainstorm. Within days after the downpour, the terrain was dotted with green plants, many of which bloomed during the next week or so. It was as though nature has stood waiting for the rain; it meant the growth and blossoming of plants that had learned to hoard the seeds of survival until the next downpour.

Environmental conditions contribute to the thriving of a life form, to the stunting of growth and the shortening of life, or, as in the case of the dinosaur, to ultimate extinction. Survival ethics grow from a recognition of the innate drive toward survival, which is found in every living organism. In and of itself, that drive is neither good nor bad, moral nor immoral; it simply is.

At its most primitive level, survival may be conceived in terms of nature "red in tooth and claw" or as the survival of the fittest. However these notions may be interpreted, it is amply clear that from most ancient times to today, survival among more highly developed life forms requires cooperation between parent and progeny (especially in such species as *Homo sapiens* where the newborn is helpless and vulnerable). For humans, at least, social cooperation is essential for the vitalization of existence (see chapter 16 on loneliness).

Survival ethics are concerned with the principles that protect life and ensure continuation. They have evolved from the fact that, in the struggle for survival, most living creatures seek to protect the lives of mates and offspring, at least until progeny can fend for themselves. Protective social patterns vary. At maturation, wild animals become self-sufficient and seek their own food, shelter, protection, and mate(s). Some creatures operate in packs or herds with which they guarantee the security of the group and share the results of the search for food and water. Within this drive to survive, different familial patterns have evolved. For example, in some species the female has sexual relationships with numerous males and by virtue of this anonymity of fatherhood she ensures the presence of male protection for herself and her offspring. In another setting, a dominant male may provide leadership for the pack while jealously guarding his sexual right over the females. In still other instances, one male and one female mate for life. In each case, survival of the individual and of the group is paramount, and survival includes food, shelter (where necessary), and protection or security from predators.

Such basic data hold true for humans. Most of us live in groups that may be as small as a family or as large as a neighborhood, a town, or a city. Within the group, principles and rules operate for the protection of individuals and the entire group. Even the person who dwells alone operates within this larger context.

We testify to our belief in survival as a basic value in the present efforts made to protect, extend, and prolong life. Beneficial survival efforts are those that maximize the potential for the individual and the group to exist physically, mentally, and spiritually at the highest, noblest, and safest levels. Just how each of these levels might be interpreted can vary from society to society, but in terms of our present human development, a democratic society provides the greatest opportunity for the highest expression of survival ethics and is to be preferred over state control or dictatorship, no matter how benevolent.

Some would go so far as to argue that the sacralization of life is the key to the most beneficial survival ethic, but much would depend upon whether life was defined as sacred because it represents the creation of some deity or whether life is to be recognized environmentally as sacred because it, like everything else in the cosmos, is a special though not yet fully understood component of the universe. This is not to imply that there is any ultimate meaning to existence—human or otherwise—but rather, to suggest that because we humans value it, life is given meaning and deemed precious (see chapter 10 on meaning). Thus survival itself is worthy of ethical consideration.

HEALTH AND SURVIVAL

Progress in living standards has contributed to the creation of numerous health benefits that extend life for humans. Diseases and plagues that once killed children or decimated populations have, for the most part, been controlled. Sanitation regulations and other public health measures guard the well-being of the general populace. Pharmaceutical research, nutrition programs, bioengineering, medical diagnosis, and technology serve to both protect humans from life-threatening diseases and contribute to longevity. In other words, human survival has benefited from efforts to improve health and engender longer lives. Obviously, not all diseases are under control and, from time to time, new epidemics appear.

Some facets of human progress can be recognized as expressions of disdain for life and a denial of the sacredness concept. Industrial and chemical technology contribute to the pollution of the atmosphere, the soil, and the water. In some areas, the environment has been so negatively affected that despite advances in modern health patterns, pollution has devastated the health of children and shortened the life span of adults. Until enforceable laws are enacted, the fouling of the environment will continue and, consequently, the lives of future adult populations will be burdened with the effects of today's pollution.

Governmental response to health threats is not always rational. For example, on the one hand, governmental health authorities warn the populace of the danger of heart disease, cancer, and a multitude of associated illnesses related to cigarette smoking. On the other hand, the same government protects and underwrites the growing of tobacco for the manufacture of these health-and life-destroying products.

The licensing of the sale of alcohol was designed to eliminate profits for the criminal underworld who bootlegged illicit liquor. However, this same licensing resulted in an increase in alcohol consumption, the swelling of numbers of alcohol addicts, and the consequent social problems stemming from alcohol abuse including drunken brutality and the destruction of families, disruption of work patterns, and so forth. In addition, there are numerous health problems stemming from the consumption of alcohol.

Present efforts to control the sale of illegal drugs elicit social pressure for the legalization of the sale of addictive narcotics. If we are to learn from the legislation related to the sale of alcohol, the effort to control crime associated with drugs through legalization may increase drug use and drug addiction with the consequent social, economic, familial, and personal health problems. Meanwhile, little is done to meet the personal and social crises that lead people of every class, race, religion, and social status to seek escape in narcotic stupor.

SURVIVAL NEEDS

Beyond environmental and health issues are the needs for food, clothing, shelter, and security. The fulfillment of these needs varies with societal patterns. A student from Beijing, China, was confused at the sight of hundreds of men and women living on skid row; barely surviving on food and clothing handouts from charitable organizations, sleeping in abandoned buildings, in cheap hotels, or on the streets; vulnerable to violence; without work and without hope or anticipation of change. As she became aware of the slow but inevitable disintegration of the psyches of these people, her confusion grew. How could one of the richest and most powerful nation in the world permit such conditions to exist? What hope for the future was there for the children of skid row? She acknowledged the absence of affluence in Communist China, where food tended to be simple and sometimes scarce, clothing standardized, and housing humble, but in China there were no street people, no elders probing the depths of garbage bins looking for scraps of food or for aluminum cans to be recycled for money to buy bread. In her homeland, food, clothing and shelter, however limited, were available for all. What had happened to the societal patterns in America that resulted in the evolution of a class of humans for whom the satisfaction of the basic needs of survival were reduced to such primitive levels? Which society had developed the highest form of survival ethics?

Most elders, we are told, live above the poverty level. Of these, many exist on the thin border that places them barely beyond the poverty level. They live in fear and insecurity, troubled by the rising prices of food, clothing, and shelter. Their survival is threatened. They know that a single tragic accident or illness could strip them of the little that they have. They have arrived at that place where they are not poor enough to qualify for public aid, not rich enough to feel secure. They live within their means—just making it. They have bought no new clothes for years. Some purchase the discards of others from thrift shops. They are restricted in their movements because travel costs, even by bus in their local communities, are high. Their pleasures are limited to what they can enjoy free of charge. Some live close enough to senior citizen centers to take advantage of social activities provided there. Others depend on friends, neighbors, and relatives to enrich their existence with visits and conversation.

For those below the poverty level, life is reduced to a day-by-day struggle to exist. We see them with their illegally acquired shopping carts loaded with their few worldly possessions. We know that most will be short-lived. Some will die from exposure; others will be beaten, raped, and murdered. They have no warm homes to go to, no warm baths to clean their bodies, no laundry facilities to wash their clothes. Their looks portray what they are—beaten down, crushed, defeated, hopeless discards.

Among these outcasts are elders who helped America and other first world countries achieve the strength, the power, and the richness that mark their affluence. Among them are those who farmed until drought caused them to leave the land and who then labored at menial tasks until their energy and strength gave out or they were replaced by younger men and women who will one day become the indigent elders of the future. Some, the handymen who could fix almost anything, have been replaced by men and women with better and more specialized training. Some elders are women who raised families as single mothers and who worked as servants in the homes of others or who took low-paying jobs to sustain their families. Often their children have moved to other parts of the world and have abandoned them. Some are aged parents with inadequately trained children who are in straits as desperate as the elders. Still other elders are absolutely alone, with no living family to inquire about their well-being. Food, clothing, shelter, protection—the basic requirements for survival—consist of whatever is available.

Even as we voice our belief in the importance of life, liberty, and the pursuit of happiness, and as we pour funds into disease-eradicating and life-extending research, we fail to provide resources that will assure healthful, decent standards of living for the poor elderly among us. Nor is any attention given to meaningful social roles for elders. We dismiss the rich supply of wisdom, talent, and diverse qualities possessed by these persons.

Who is responsible for protecting the elders? Our society is a strange mixture of individual responsibility and cooperative living for the benefit of the person, the group, the community, the state, the nation, and, ultimately, the world. Unlike our most ancient migratory ancestors, most of us no longer forage for food and build temporary shelters when needed. We live in communities where we assume communal responsibilities for our own and our neighbor's safety and well-being. Our children are raised to be independent, to seek meaningful employment and to provide for themselves. Those of us who don't make it enter the ranks of the unwanted, the unloved and disposable.

Some elders, through inheritance or through profitable earnings can protect their own well-being by purchasing the best in living conditions and health protection. Their self-esteem is protected and can only be diminished by increasing physical fragility assuming that mental processes are still healthy.

For the rest, the government becomes more and more the means of guaranteeing survival, of protecting health, and of maintaining feelings of self-worth. Of course, historical records testify to the numerous ways in which governments have botched their responsibilities by devising inadequate (even repelling) settings and situations that have deprived individuals and classes of people of civil rights or the right to live. Even when the government acts on behalf of poorer citizens, the outreach bears negative labels such as "welfare" or "relief" that can humiliate and demean by implying that recipients are failures.

A government, functioning at its best, provides a social system that assures individuals a sense of personal worth: no matter how menial the task performed or how high-sounding the office, people know that their work contributes significantly and in ways that truly matter to the betterment of the whole. Our present social structure teaches that money and power count most. Therefore the individual can only measure personal worth or significance in terms of these two criteria. Then, what happens to values such as courage, love, integrity, fair play? We acknowledge their importance by momentary recognition of individuals or in large scale programs that we label "Fair Deal" politics or the policies of "The Great Society."

Survival ethics raises a fundamental human and personal question: To whom does the individual belong? As far back as we can go in history we find differing answers. From religion comes the answer: to God. According to this way of thinking, we are "creatures of God" and the purpose of our lives on earth is to fulfill the divine will, either by praising the deity or by living according to divinely revealed regulations. Government has answered that we belong to the state or the community. Our responsibilities are tied to the welfare of the state, and as the state prospers so does the individual. Industrial enterprises might provide a different response by claiming that individuals belong to the company for whom they work, since it is through job identity that the person is able to declare who she or he is. Familial responsibilities suggest that we belong to the family of which we are a part. The bonding that marks that identity begins at birth and is reenforced by dependency through childhood. Mature adults might argue that they belong only to the self, arguing that if life does not belong to the self then it has no personal meaning.

Ethical systems tend to embrace multiple belongings. The person belongs to himself or herself as an individual and of course the primary responsibility to the self is preservation. However, the ethic that stresses survival of self may be compromised by familial bonds, by religious affiliations, and by national awareness. History is littered with accounts of self-sacrifice for others, particularly for members of the family or for others whom one loves. For example, religious causes sparked the Jonestown deaths, where members of the cult died by their own hand for their faith, and millions of lives have been lost in wars for the sake of the nation. In other words, an ethic that stresses only personal survival may falter in the face of one that embraces a wider constituency.

Who determines when the survival ethic extends beyond the person? In time of military struggle, the personal survival of youth is sacrificed on the altar of Mars (the god of war). In business, the well-being of the individual may be sacrificed on the altar of profit. In the family, the good of one person may be set aside in favor of the needs of the group.

How do these patterns affect elders? We have learned that when the thin veneer of civilization is stripped away, as it was in Nazi Germany, the handicapped and the elderly can be done away with for the good of the state. If they cannot produce, they do not deserve to eat and live. Germany was recognized as one of the most civilized of nations—a people that had produced great humanitarians, great poets and musicians, and great religious leaders. But in a spasm of history, the survival ethic underwent dramatic change, and elders became members of groups slated for the death camps. Their existence had ceased to have meaning.

Religions that mouth slogans concerning the importance of human life and of respect for the elderly have forsaken their humanistic ethic and have found ways to destroy life, particularly the lives of the disadvantaged and the old in everything from witchcraft trials to holy wars. No concern is expressed for the aged in the battles of Northern Ireland nor in the conflicts in Lebanon, where Christian blows up Christian and Muslim cuts down Muslim without respect for age. Indeed, some of those most vulnerable to the dishonest activities of an unscrupulous minority of church leaders have been the aged who trusted these so-called men and women of God to handle their funds with respect and care, only to be left disenchanted if not completely destitute.

Clearly, business has no vested interest in elder care. A given organization may have a retirement plan, but once the employee has retired there is no more interest in that person; he or she no longer contributes to company income. Some corporations have health-care programs that can be continued by the employee but most companies don't. Retirees are on their own.

Nor does the family always care for elders. As we shall see in the discussion of elder abuse (chapter 7), the greatest violation of personal safety and care is perpetrated by family members.

WHO, THEN, IS RESPONSIBLE FOR THE ELDERS?

At present both the family and the state have acknowledged responsibility: the former for reasons of bonding, loyalty, social pressure, and guilt; the latter because society has insisted that the state assume a moral stance concerning the welfare of all of its citizens. Most of us are decent, caring human beings. At the same time, in periods of stress, something less than respect for others can be manifested. As costs for the long-term care of elders continues to mount, we are beginning to hear the voices of those who see themselves as "practical" politicians call for limiting services to elders and suggesting that older adults need to get out of the way of youth. Already in families where financial and job stress are present, frail elders can become nuisances and burdens that the family resents.

It is obvious that, *ideally,* the first line of defense for the protection of elders is the family; *practically,* however, the first line will have to be governmental services. The recognition of elder contributions to the development of a society places ethical demands on that society to provide for the basic survival needs of its elders. Perhaps this demand requires an increase in taxation, and the establishing of government insured retirement programs to which employers and employees contribute throughout a lifetime (like an Individual Retirement Account). Any such programs must be designed to guard against economic inflation and depression, and provide guarantees for the acquisition of adequate food, clothing, shelter, and health services.

At the same time, families and individuals must be taught to provide for themselves by looking ahead to the time when those who are now young will become elders. Most of us simply drift into old age. How many depression kids gave thought to becoming elderly? Some did and they are presently protected by their own investments. Most did not, and their numbers swell the ranks of dependent elders whose plight so frustrates some politicians.

We who are advocates for elder protection must present a twofold platform. One plank will be concerned with the immediate situation, with the growing number of elders who need help *now.* The second plank will represent the future, so that when the middle aged and young become elders they will be assured of proper care for their survival needs. If present needs require that taxes be raised, then so be it. *We are responsible for one another.* What is even more pressing in the United States is the immediate development of a national health insurance program. If long-range plans for the protection of future elders requires individual contributions to a protective fund, then such a program must incorporate employees, employers, and governmental taxation, and it must be developed now.

The issue is not that we are ruled by "extravagant expectations," to use Daniel J. Boorstin's phrase; we are truly a practical people (Boorstin 1962, p. 4). We are concerned with basic survival needs. We do not ask or demand or even expect more than our fair shake, which includes the privilege of growing old without the burden of fear and worry about how we are to survive.

SURVIVAL, HEALTH, AND MEANING

Health and meaning are given separate treatment in this book (chapters 14 and 7 respectively), but both are significant when discussing ways in which elders confront survival in the face of illnesses that have been diagnosed as, or that appear to be, terminal. There are those who argue that mindset, attitude, and mode of confronting or dealing with life-threatening conditions contribute to what some view as "miraculous" escapes from the grim reaper.

The relationship of the mind to the body has long been recognized and heatedly discussed. More than twenty-five years ago, Dr. William Nolen conducted a study of so-called faith healing (cf. Larue 1990, pp. 114–74). He commented:

> Some patients, admittedly lose that impossible-to-define but very real spirit we call "the will to live." These patients, usually very sick, elderly people, don't actually seek death, but they refuse to cooperate in the fight to save their lives. (Nolen 1974, p. 4)

Upon recovery, the survival instinct prevails, but, Nolen continued, "often, however, without their cooperation we fight a losing battle and they die."

In recent years, a number of books and articles have been published dealing with the "holistic" approach to medicine in which attitude is linked to recovery. The "will to live" or the survival instinct motivates the energizing of the total individual to do battle against the disease. Arnold Hutschnecker recorded the story of an elderly woman who recalled that at middle age she suffered a life-threatening illness. He describes how she rallied her resources:

> She lay hovering between life and death, in the twilight of half-surrender, . . . she overheard two of her co-workers talking just outside the open door of her hospital room.
>
> "If we could only reach her! If we could only make her understand," one of them said passionately, "how much we need her!" (Hutschnecker 1954, p. 52)

He goes on to say, "In a moment of discouragement and wavering faith, the intensity of her colleague's plea reassured her and gave her the courage to take up the struggle again" (p. 54). In other words, if one has something to live for, the will to survive contributes to recovery and health.

Sudden reversals of illnesses, some of which have been diagnosed as terminal, are not uncommon in medicine. What causes or triggers the healing is not always known or understood, but something in the psyche and the body musters the person's survival resources and the illness is defeated. The holistic concept of medicine suggests that a mind-body relationship is at work.

Of course, the will to live, the determination to survive does not always work. Virginia Hine's *Last Letter to the Pebble People* (1979) records the heroic struggle of Alden Hine to slow or defeat inoperable lung cancer employing hope, love, faith, and prayer. Nothing really worked, not even the support network of people who each day set aside ten or fifteen minutes to concentrate on Alden in the vain hope of somehow magically transferring energy to the ailing man. After fifteen months Alden died what is described as a "victorious death," despite the fact that the will-to-live and the encouragement of others did not overcome the ravages of the disease.

The relationship between survival and having something to live for that gives meaning to existence is well-documented from concentration camp experiences. Bruno Bettelheim (1979), writing out of his personal experiences in Nazi concentration camps at Dachau and Buchenwald in 1938, argued that "to survive, one had to want to survive for a purpose" (p. 293), otherwise "if one gave up hope, one lost the ability to go on with the difficult and painful struggle survival required and so one died in a short time" (p. 106).

Loss of will-to-live may occur when elders are placed in nursing homes against their will. The transition marks the abandonment of a familiar environment endowed with personal belongings that have meaning to a setting where few personal items are allowed. Nursing homes function according to schedules. The loss of personal freedom to live according to one's own preferred patterns signifies not only the loss of the right to choose for ones self but dependency on what others have decided. Many families have remarked on the changes in personality and physical appearance of elders shortly after they enter a nursing home. Perhaps the elder is affected by awareness that the nursing home is where he or she has gone to die. Perhaps loneliness in a strange environment is a contributing factor. Inactivity may also add to the "flat" affect or the lack of any emotion in response to life. Awareness that his or her care has become too much of a responsibility for even the most loving family to handle reminds the elder that he or she has become a burden to those who matter most. It is not surprising that the death trajectory can become accelerated for sensitive older persons.

ENHANCING THE WILL-TO-LIVE

If survival ethics embraces the societal wish to enhance life for elders and to help sustain the will-to-live, what steps can be taken to actualize these concerns? One immediately thinks of local programs and activities sponsored by community centers and churches. There can be no question that these are important in the lives of some elders, but they do not help older adults in nursing homes or those confined to their own homes because of physical handicaps.

Some of the housebound have stated that the persons who deliver meals-on-wheels or who come to help with house cleaning are their only contacts with the outside world. Neither of these sources of assistance provides any touching or physical contact, which can be so important in reassuring the elder that he or she has not become one of the world's untouchables. Case workers are overburdened and can do little more than make occasional visits. The result can be ever-deepening depression. Some churches have volunteer visitors for their members, but the elderly who lack church affiliation are not included in parochial outreach programs. Perhaps volunteers could be trained to assist case workers by making regular visits to shut-ins, after the fashion of the hospice program volunteers.

Out of necessity, nursing homes provide some physical contact, and the professional touch is better than none at all. What resident elders need are gestures of caring that provide reassurance of their importance in the eyes of the caregivers. Nursing home programs that go beyond placing patients in front of a television set and involve them in creative expressions alleviate feelings of uselessness and enhance the will-to-live.

Survival ethics are expressions of human concern for other humans to the end that the will-to-live is strengthened no matter what the social situation.

REFERENCES

Bettelheim, Bruno. 1979. *Surviving (and Other Essays)*. New York: Alfred A. Knopf.

Boorstin, Daniel J. 1962. *The Image, or What Happened to the American Dream*. New York: Atheneum.

Cousins, Norman. 1983. *The Healing Heart: Antidotes to Panic and Help-lessness*. New York: W. W. Norton and Company.

Hine, Virginia. 1977, 1979. *Last Letter to the Pebble People.* Santa Cruz, Calif.: Unity Press.

Hutschnecker, Arnold A. 1954. *The Will to Live.* Garden City, N.Y.: Permabooks.

Larue, Gerald A. 1990. *The Supernatural, the Occult, and the Bible.* Buffalo, N.Y.: Prometheus Books.

Nolen, William A. 1974. *Healing: A Doctor in Search of a Miracle.* New York: Random House.

Pelletier, Kenneth R. 1977. *Mind as Healer, Mind as Slayer: A Holistic Approach to Preventing Stress Disorders.* New York: Dell Publishing Co.

6

Elder Power

"As 'the elders of the tribe' and professionals in aging, we must prepare ourselves to challenge oppressive powers by continuing analysis of their policies and systems, confronting them with the social consequences of what they do with their own forgotten humanity."

—Margaret E. Kuhn, "What Old People
Want for Themselves," pp. 93–94

Elder power refers to the potential political and societal influence that can be exercised by elders in present time and in the near future. Elder power can affect legislation relating to the welfare and well-being of older persons throughout the community. When their security is threatened, elders can use their power to move beyond party loyalty to support or oppose legislation that bears on this vital concern. Protests can change the way elders are portrayed in the media. Reporting potentially threatening situations can call attention to abuse and neglect of elders, thereby raising social awareness and enhancing the likelihood of change.

Many elders are beginning to recognize themselves as members of a very special age group consisting of those who during a lifetime have paid their dues to society and who now should be able to reap benefits for services rendered, whether given in part or in full. They now share a body of common concerns, particularly those relating to physical and economic security as well as health issues. Many live in retirement communities or housing projects designed for the elderly where meeting places provide potential forums for the discussion of elder issues. Others gather at public recreation centers. Some thirty-two million belong to The

American Association of Retired Persons (AARP) and regularly receive copies of *Modern Maturity* magazine, which reports on legislation and other issues relating to elder welfare.

When Congress discusses budget reform that includes cut-backs in Social Security or Medicare, elder power reacts. Those over sixty-five years of age, who constitute only 12 percent of the population, flood congressional offices with protests that are often heeded because elders are active at the polls. In presidential elections, the elderly cast about 20 percent of the votes (Rosenblatt and Reynolds 1990).

But elder power extends beyond its own age group. Many have children who are concerned about their parents' welfare. Cutbacks in Social Security payments or in medical services threaten to place greater burdens on the children for parental care. Threatened elders pass their troubled feelings on to family members who in turn add to the protests against any legislation curtailing benefits to the elderly. Moreover, as the number of elders increases during the next decade, elder power will increase accordingly.

There can be no question that the costs of elder care are rising. In 1971, Social Security paid out 81.2 billion dollars in benefits and Medicare paid out 22.5 billion dollars; the expenditures for 1990 are 192.8 billion dollars for Social Security and 93 billion dollars for Medicare. Individual monthly payments of $571 for a single person and $970 for a couple are not large but they keep millions from abject poverty. In 1959, poverty among the elderly was 35.2 percent; in 1990 it was 12 percent. Some older persons have supplemental income in the form of retirement payments or investments, and many own their own homes. In fact, married couples between the ages of sixty-five and seventy-five are reported to enjoy the highest standard of living. Nevertheless, 29 million elders earn less than $15,000 per year; the median for men in 1989 was $13,107 and for women $7,656. The greatest poverty is among older widows—those over the age of eighty. At this level, every increase in Social Security benefits assumes immense proportions and every increase in personal payments for Medicare become impossible economic burdens (Rosenblatt and Reynolds 1990).

Of course, there are upper-income and some very wealthy persons (including some millionaires) who receive Social Security payments. Obviously, they do not need this income to survive, but through the years they have contributed their share to the fund and legally the money is theirs. To begin to draw lines and to introduce some sort of economic triage to Social Security will simply bog the system down in more bureaucratic red tape and add more confusion to a system already overloaded with paper work. In addition, when the Congress, whose members are already well paid both in salary and perquisites, continually vote themselves immense increases in salary, efforts to cut back on Social Security and to add costs to those who use Medicare appear both hypocritical and undemocratic. Elder power may not be able to rescind the benefits claimed by elected representatives, but it can put a damper on tampering with Social Security and Medicare.

There are those who are fearful that by the year 2005 Social Security funds, which are today in good shape, will be drained because of the increasing demands by the growing number of elders, particularly when the so-called baby-boomers reach sixty-five years of age. Some question the wisdom of contributing money that they may never get back. They wonder whether they would be better off by investing in some private system to guard against poverty in old age. The baby-boomers' fears are not unfounded. Quite often there is anger at being compelled to contribute to a retirement program that may not pay back what has been invested. Nevertheless, the nation must have in hand a plan that protects the elderly from poverty. If and when national health insurance is enacted, some relief will be given to Social Security funds. Moreover, those whose health will be protected from infancy throughout life will be healthier elders who may wish to remain in productive work beyond the usual times for retirement. The declining birth rate may reduce the potential work force so that the demand for workers to fill needed jobs may make elders eligible for meaningful employment well into what would have been their retirement years. At present there is no good answer to the troubled baby-boomers; elders simply do their best. Elders, on the other hand, seek to protect the fund from those legislators who eye the immense reserve and seek to tap it for other projects.

It should not be assumed that elders are opposed to increases in taxes. What is opposed is unequal increases. When the very rich pay less in taxes than those in the middle-income groups in which many elders find themselves, the unfairness of the tax system raises protests. Increased taxes on products used by poor and near-poor elders saps their spirit of hope. Younger poor and near-poor persons may entertain hope for surcease by looking to employment or better jobs in the future. No such hope exists for elders, the majority of whom are unemployable with incomes that are severely limited.

While elder power serves to protect the interests and concerns of the elderly, there is the ever-present danger of a backlash from those who may feel somehow disenfranchised by the power of elder voting. For example, in cases where school bonds have been voted down because elders in the community do not feel obliged to pay for new schools inasmuch as they have no children to be served, parents feel cheated. Their efforts to provide the best education for their children have been thwarted by a power group who appears to have no concern for either the present or the future of young people. Of course, there are elders who are deeply concerned about the education of young people. Their vote against tax increases to finance new schools reflects the insecurity of those whose income is limited and who cannot hope for the increases that young job holders anticipate as they mature in their employment. Their negative vote symbolizes a preoccupation with survival: elders versus the young. Such situations can only breed tensions.

Backlash may come in the form of a self-imposed agism or in the segregation of elders. Cluster voting can produce an image of older persons as a separate group, opposed to certain forms of progress, interested only in their own well-being, and therefore to be considered apart from younger and perhaps mainstream life. This leads to segregated thinking and living.

The ethical implications are important. Neighborhoods have been known to split apart over such antagonism. Where there is anger and frustration there is potential for tapping reservoirs of violence. To prevent conflicts, it has been suggested that the property taxes of elders be frozen thereby freeing them from the threat of increased taxes when bond issues are proposed. This may or may not be the most viable solution, but until steps are taken to protect elder income and simultaneously free communities to act to improve education or streets or lighting or whatever, tensions will remain and the backlash will continue as a real possibility.

Elder dollars are also potent instruments affecting responses to the needs of older persons. As the number of elders grew, sales experts and advertisers channeled some of their skills to respond to this potential market. Clothing for elders moved away from the rather dowdy dresses and colors once deemed suitable for aging women and men to smart, styled, and very up-to-date garments modelled by trim, svelte, attractive elders. The marketing of health and beauty products once aimed at youth, broadened to include older men and women. Auto sales pitches, most of which pictured young television or movie beauties in sleek sports cars, now included elders—not in the square, boxlike cars most were perceived to drive, but zooming around in sleek new production models that told viewers "This is not your father's Oldsmobile." Recording companies market tape cassettes of "oldies but goodies" urging older viewers and listeners to rekindle memories of other days through music that had special meaning during their youth.

The influence of elder dollars has not been limited to sales. Merchants seeking these monies have sought to facilitate elder needs. Washrooms in shopping malls, once located down dark flights of stairs or in inaccessible corners, now provide easy access. Doors swing open easily without the need to turn knobs; and where entries and exits do utilize fastening gear, bar handles replace the slippery, hard-to-turn round fixtures that were once standard.

Homebuilders have also become aware of the importance of servicing the special needs of elders. Many now automatically build in grab bars in showers and bathtubs and next to toilets. Benches and nonslip flooring in showers and tubs are safety features that benefit everyone.

Even as we recognize the benefits that have come from the pressure exercised by elders to make their presence and their needs known, the question of the ethics of such pressures must be addressed. Is it right or fair or decent for a consortium of elders to use their voting and purchasing clout to bring about social changes that focus primarily on their particular needs, wishes, and benefits? To the degree that such legislation or changes imposes genuine hardships on others, and produces unnecessary handouts to elders, they must be challenged. So far, this has not been the pattern. On the other hand, the "forgotten humanity" that Margaret E. Kuhn refers to in the epigram to this chapter reminds us that without protests and demands for recognition by elders and their families, changes that are beneficial to all would probably not come about. Moreover, the humanitarian results of elder pressure today become the inheritance of those who will become elders in the years ahead. The insistence on the recognition of elder rights and elder needs are the legitimate demands of those living in democratic societies and, therefore, they fall well within the boundaries of ethical behavior. Voices must continue to call for recognition of the presence of elders in a society that can all too readily try to forget them.

REFERENCES

Atchley, Robert C. 1972. *The Social Forces in Later Life.* Belmont, Calif.: Wadsworth Publishing Company.

Gelfand, Donald E. 1984. *The Aging Network: Program and Services.* New York: Springer Publishing Company.

Kerschner, Paul A., ed. 1976. *Advocacy and Age.* Los Angeles: University of Southern California Press.

Kuhn, Margaret E. 1976. "What Old People Want for Themselves," in

Paul A. Kerschner, ed., *Advocacy and Age*. Los Angeles: University of Southern California Press, pp. 87–96.

Morris, Robert. 1985. *Social Policy of the American Welfare State*. New York: Longman, Inc.

Rosenblatt, Robert A., and Maura Reynolds. 1990. "Nation's Elderly Can Exert a Lot of Muscle," *The Los Angeles Times,* October 19.

7

Elder Abuse

"Unless there is widespread understanding of the phenomenon of elder abuse and neglect and society makes a commitment to a wide range of reform and assistance in both government and the private sector, the abuse, exploitation, and suffering will continue."

—Quinn and Tomita, *Elder Abuse and Neglect,* p. 6

Elder abuse, like all other forms of abuse, is dependent upon the vulnerability of the victim. Frail, lonely, and trusting elders, become high-risk victims, pawns in the hands of unscrupulous caregivers and others who would prey upon them. This troubling national problem, whose frequency, at present, appears to be only slightly below that of child abuse, is expected to worsen as the population of elders in our society increases. The number of cases of elder abuse remains unknown. Present studies suggest that some four percent of elders, about one million per year, are abused, but it is estimated that only one out of six cases is reported, inasmuch as many elders have no way to assert their rights and some lack the physical and mental capability to present their cases. In addition, many professionals and paraprofessionals who would ordinarily record abuses have not been adequately trained in recognizing the signs of elder abuse (Quinn and Tomita 1986, p. 2).

WHAT IS ELDER ABUSE?

Elder abuse refers to the maltreatment of persons age sixty-five or older. The ill-use assumes many forms including neglect, verbal harassment, physical attacks, psychological assault, financial exploitation, and violation of civil and human rights.

Neglect

Neglect can be classified as either "passive" or "active." Passive neglect occurs when, out of caregiver ignorance or perhaps because of stress in the family or institution, needed services are not provided or are withheld from frail or dependent elders. Active neglect takes place when the omissions are deliberate and designed to hurt the older person.

The results of neglect can be devastating; reports of extreme cases of neglect in family settings shock and horrify social workers. Frail elders, unable to prepare their own food, are dependent upon whatever nourishment the caregiver provides. For example, an eighty-year-old woman lived in a remodelled garage at the back of her son's home. When the social workers investigated they found that the two-room residence was dirty and smelly. Food remnants were scattered on the floor. The toilet was plugged with paper and feces. The odors were unbearable. The woman was unkempt, unbathed, haggard, and confused. Failure to provide adequate food and water had resulted in malnutrition and dehydration. The door of the structure was kept locked from the outside because the son feared that the elderly woman might wander and become lost. For entertainment there was a television that, at best, produced fuzzy pictures.

In another case, frail grandparents, who continued to live in their own home, were confined to a locked attic room by their eldest son. Care for the aged couple was assigned to a grandson who had his own agenda. The food and liquids he brought to them were purchased at fast food outlets and were delivered on an irregular basis. Fortunately, the room had a sink and toilet so the elderly couple were able to maintain some sort of personal hygiene. Social workers investigated at the insistance of neighbors who had been friends of the elders for many years and who were concerned at not seeing them. The social workers found that the attic room was far too hot for comfort, and cockroaches were everywhere. The couple were emaciated, in declining health, frightened, and bewildered by their imprisonment. Their son argued that they were "O.K." and that because they were not being starved or beaten there was no cause for legal intervention. He said his parents had been placed in the locked attic because they might be a danger to themselves if they were permitted the run of their own home or access to the yard and street. The grandson admitted that he found his responsibilities to be a "drag" on his day, but saw no reason to question the quality or the quantity of food he brought to his elders. The family saw "nothing wrong" with the situation and felt that the neighbors and the social workers were butting into something that did not concern them! Unfortunately, such accounts of mistreated elders abound.

In poorly run and understaffed nursing homes busy ward aides ignore the special needs of patients. Some elders require extended periods of time for eating that the caregiver may not be willing to give; consequently food and beverages are removed before the elder has finished eating. Clients who are too weak to reach for a glass of water must wait until the caregiver responds. If an elder has bladder problems, liquids may be withhold to reduce the need to change clothing or bed linen. Sunken eyes and cheeks, extreme thirst, weight loss, confusion, apathy, and perhaps hallucinations are all symptoms of such neglect.

Neglect may involve ignoring the need of bedridden elders to have their position changed regularly. Prolonged pressure on soft tissues inhibits adequate blood supply causing pressure sores on the bony parts of the body such as elbows, heels, and hips. These sores, that begin as reddened areas, rapidly progress to blisters and then to open sores that can become infected, causing permanent damage and even death.

Neglect also includes failure to assist in personal hygiene. Patients who are unable to clean and bathe themselves are simply ignored. Failure to provide essential medical care for physical or mental needs is a form of neglect as well. In some instances, safety hazards are ignored and elders suffer unnecessary injuries.

Psychological Abuse

Psychological abuse produces mental anguish ranging from shame, confusion, disorientation, fear of talking about certain subjects, and at times even attempts at suicide. As Erich Fromm (1973) has pointed out, "Mental sadism may be disguised in many seemingly harmless ways: a question, a smile, a confusing remark" (p. 284). Victims can be humiliated and made to feel inadequate because of their inability to function on their own. They can be ridiculed for physical ineptness, or mocked and made to feel guilt if they drop or spill food. The elderly can be bullied and harassed, intimidated and threatened by everything from name calling to being shouted at in bursts of anger until they become fearful for their safety. Many elders are quite vulnerable and so can be manipulated by being denied information or by being given false or confusing information, by being forced to depend on the will of others in everything from making a phone call to spending money. The name of the game is "control," through which the abuser assumes power over the elder(s).

Financial Abuse

Financial or fiduciary abuses range from outright theft of the elder's assets and the bilking of small amounts of money through fradulent schemes to the acquisition of deeds to property. Sometimes personal belongings—including art, jewelry, and clothing—are stolen or taken and sold to support a drug habit. An elderly widow living in filthy conditions, not eating, not taking her medicines, unbathed, and wearing dirty clothes was bilked out of $25,000 by a neighbor woman and her son who had assumed the role of caretakers. They had persuaded the eighty-six-year-old woman that she had financial problems and had to sell her car, stocks, and finally her home (to them) at a price far below market value. They even wrote checks on her bank account. The confused and abused elder was rescued after her plight was reported to local officials.

Attentive bankers may became concerned when there is unusual activity in an elder's account, when large sums are withdrawn from savings, when bank statements and cancelled checks are ordered to be sent to an address other than the elder's home. On the other hand, bankers can be abusers—as became obvious with the failure of various savings and loans when it was disclosed that many elders were reduced to poverty because they had been deceived into believing that the bonds they were persuaded to purchase through these institutions were covered by federal deposit insurance. Indeed, so severe was the impact of loss that at least one elderly investor, having lost his life savings, committed suicide (Connelly 1990).

Fiscal abuse can also be inflicted by ruthless sales persons who engage in fraudulent business practices. Some use the telephone, others go door to door in communities with high concentrations of elders to persuade these persons to have driveways refinished, to purchase fiberglass burial containers (Jain 1990), to have house numbers painted on their roof tops to assist helicopter police patrols, or to buy equipment that the elder does not need and in some cases cannot use. Often when services are provided the products used are inferior: for example, the numbers on various roof tops were washed away by the first rain, and the driveway coating was in some cases just a thin covering of water-based paint.

Physical Abuse

Physical abuse refers to intentional, malicious acts that inflict physical injuries ranging from bruises and scratches to sprains, burns, abrasions, fractures, dislocations, welts, internal injuries, sexual assaults, and even death. Medical personnel become alerted to physical mistreatment when they find old, healing bruises together with new contusions signifying repeated injury. Sometimes rope burns and pressure sores at ankles, wrists, and under the arms indicate forced confinement to a chair or a bed over long periods of time. Some have reported finding bald spots where chunks of hair had been forcibly jerked from an elder's head. Physical abuse, particularly in nursing homes, includes the use of restraints when patients are tied down in lieu of proper treatment.

Medicinal abuse occurs both in poorly supervised nursing homes and in the family setting. Chemical restraint, which of course means sedation, is employed to keep elders compliant and subdued.

Sexual abuses, which can have the most devastating effects on elders, include battery (the touching or fondling of an intimate part of the elder), rape, incest, sodomy, oral copulation, and penetration of genital and anal openings by foreign objects. The damage resulting from these abuses affect body, mind, and spirit, for the elder has been reduced to the status of an object to be used rather than treated as a human to be respected and cherished. Consequently, sexually abused elders suffer pain and infections, and often become fearful, depressed, and confused. As feelings of helplessness and hopelessness increase, their vitality and spirit almost disappear. The physical and verbal examinations that follow reported sexual abuse can add to feelings of humiliation and be upsetting to the elder, evoking memories of what was felt during the assaults. Some elders are troubled by concern about how family members may react to this particular kind of abuse; others express insecurity about their futures.

WHO ARE THE ABUSED?

Data identifying exactly which elders are most likely to be victimized are imprecise. A recent study by Karl Pillemer and David Finkelhor found:

Interestingly, the rates of abuse and neglect were no higher for minority
than for white elderly, no higher for older (over 75) than for younger
(64–74) elderly, and not significantly different for those of any religious,
economic or educational background. (1988, p. 54)

In addition, they found that elder spouse abuse was approximately equal
to that of children abusing their elderly parents, and that men were equally
likely to be victims of spousal abuse (p. 54). On a broader level, their
findings did not demonstrate that women rather than men were more
likely to be victims of elder abuse; in fact, "the risk of abuse for elderly
men is double that of elderly women," although because there are fewer
elderly men, the numbers of abused elderly women and men were about
the same (p. 55).

The above findings are in sharp contrast to earlier studies, which claimed
that the most typical victim of elder abuse was likely to be a single female,
over age seventy-five, living in the home of a relative, and suffering from
some form of disability that made her extremely dependent on others.
Most were supposed to be widowed white women. These elders tended
to be financially dependent with more than 50 percent living below the
officially designated poverty level. An estimated 75 percent were believed
to have mental or physical impairments requiring costly and extensive
medical care. Obviously, such persons would feel helpless, without control over their lives, and unable to change their situations. Often, due
to physical and mental impairment, they would be socially isolated, hence
their maltreatment would not be known outside of the household. Of
course, the most recent study does not mean that some of the conditions
found by earlier investigators have no validity. What has been changed
are the estimates of which elders are most vulnerable and who the per-
petrators of abuse might be.

As we will see, the population of abused elders also includes those
who live in nursing homes and long-term care facilities. Here, too, elders
may experience situations in which they feel unable to defend themselves
or protest maltreatment.

WHO ARE THE ABUSERS?

On November 7, 1980, an article by George Mair was reprinted in the
Los Angeles Times. It began as follows:

The United States has a new indoor sport that may rest alongside incest as a forbidden subject. It is called "granny bashing" and involves adult children beating their aged parents senseless to steal the Social Security check or literally forcing mommy to eat her dinner off the floor like a dog.

The examples he cited came from testimony given before Congress and are only two of hundreds of similar or more disturbing accounts.

Most abusers in family settings live with the abused and are the victim's primary caregiver. They are the adult children of the elder: sons, daughters, daughters-in-law and sons-in-law, and, in some cases, the grandchildren. The most damaging physical abuse, including sexual abuse, is most often inflicted by sons who display sociopathic tendencies and who, although they are adults, have not reached the level of maturity that would induce them to leave home. It is estimated that 65 percent of male abusers come from homes where they were abused or in which they witnessed the abuse of their mothers (Quinn and Tomita 1986). Among the factors contributing to abuse are stress and the high degree of dependency of the elder. Alcoholism and drug abuse may also be involved.

In nursing home settings abusers are usually caretaking staff of varying status within the institution. Some were abused as children, while others see their role as nothing more than a job to be expedited with the least amount of energy or involvement in the well-being of the patients. Thus these abusers tend to become indifferent and even callous in their treatment of elders. In understaffed nursing homes, the abusers may be more concerned with control of elders than with improving the patients' quality of life, hence abuse in the form of physical and chemical restraints is not unusual.

In both private homes and in institutions caregivers, having grown weary of responsibilities, become apathetic. They look with indifference and without feeling at the sad situation of those dependent on them. Fortunately, these caregivers are not the majority.

WHO REPORTS ABUSE?

The most common reporters of elder abuse are social workers who have been trained to recognize the signs. However, because social workers may be overworked and underpaid, considerable time can elapse before in-home visits are made or residential settings are inspected.

Some reports are made by neighbors who become aware that the elder, who was once a familiar figure, is no longer seen. Sometimes they overhear sounds of brutalization. Out of concern for the elder they contact social service agencies.

On occasion, family members will report the abuse. They become so disturbed at what is happening to the dependent elder that they feel compelled to contact authorities, even though they know full well that an investigation will result in prosecution of the abusing family member.

Some find it puzzling to learn that when confronted by doctors or social workers abused elders often deny the abuse. They choose to remain in a setting that is familiar rather than be moved to an unknown environment that offers safety and security. Few elders personally report abuse, partly out of ignorance of the social system designed to protect them, partly because of the belief that there is no place of refuge available, and partly out of fear of retaliation from the abuser. Because more provisions have been made for the care of battered women, elder females who are victims of spouse abuse have shelters available, but, once again, they hesitate to leave the comparative security of the home for the insecurity of an unknown future.

It is obvious that understaffed social service departments in large cities cannot respond to all complaints immediately, and they cannot solve all problems. It has been estimated that approximately 95 percent of reported cases receive no help. Where assistance is available, neglected elders can be helped through in-home services while abused elders can be separated from their abusers.

POLICIES AND LEGISLATION

Although reporting of elder abuse is mandatory in most states, there is in the statutes a lack of uniformity that may range from the definition of abuse to response to the situation. Mandatory reporting laws require doctors, dentists, nurses, social workers, psychiatrists, chiropractors, licensed therapists, care providers, social service employees, and anyone else who works with the elderly to report cases of abuse. In some states, failure to report can result in fines. Moral and ethical concerns prompt those outside of officialdom to become involved. Reports are made to social service agencies, which then become responsible for removing the victim and arranging counseling for both the abused and the abuser.

ELDER ABUSE IN THE FAMILY SETTING

Strange as it may seem, a large percentage of elder abuse occurs in family settings. Within the family the most frequent single abuser is the son of the victim (21 percent) followed by the daughter (17 percent), then the spouse. For many, it is hard to believe that loved ones are treated so cruelly. What happens in a family to give rise to maltreatment of a frail or helpless elder? A number of factors have been recognized (Fulmer and O'Malley 1987, p. 37).

Family dynamics can produce an environment open to abuse. In some families emotional upset and anger have always found their expression in violence, or through intimidation or withdrawal. The angry person (young or old) screams and shouts, throws and breaks objects, physically assaults another, and in one way or another uses strength and destructive intent to express feelings or to force compliance. Even mere threats of violent behavior can affect another's security. The withdrawal of love and support or resorting to noncommunication, or the threat of such treatment, become weapons designed to punish, hurt, and isolate. Theories of transgenerational violence suggest that violence is learned and passed on from one generation to the next. As we have noted, it is estimated that 65 percent of male abusers come from homes in which they were abused or in which they saw their mothers abused.

Sometimes elder abuse is an expression of retaliation for past grievances—real or imagined. The controlling person wants revenge and seeks ways to even a score related to what happened in the past when the patient was in control.

In cases where family ties were never close or supportive, the need for the family to provide care for an elder becomes an unwanted, burdensome task. If financial resources are strained, the older person's dependency may be seen as an added pressure on an already overstressed family. When elder income from Social Security is incorporated as a source of family income, familial needs may take priority over those of the elder and the money may not be used to help the older member. Medical costs that exceed an elder's ability to pay place a drain on the caretaker's resources at a time when there may be other financial expenditures, such as those associated with college education of children. In these strained settings, elder abuse develops, ranging in intensity from gestures and words that make the elder feel uncomfortable or burdensome, to outright brutality.

Abusers are often under situational stress due to loss of employment, divorce, or being part of a dysfunctional family. In such cases, a frail elder can be viewed as an irritating extra nuisance, demanding time, attention, and energy. Some caregivers are addicted to alcohol and drugs and some have emotional problems and/or a history of psychiatric disturbances. Sadistic abusers are sociopathic personalities with serious emotional imbalances that make it impossible for them to form meaningful relationships with others or feel guilt for their actions. Some are mentally retarded or suffering from some chronic inability to make appropriate judgments regarding the dependent elder. It has been estimated that 31 percent of abusers have histories of psychiatric illness, and 43 percent have substance abuse problems (O'Malley et al. 1983, pp. 998–1005). Obviously such abusers confront social workers and health practitioners with unique problems. They tend to ignore the elder's basic needs including food, clothing, shelter, and medical care despite repeated intervention by authorities. Abusers have difficulty in recognizing the relationship of their behavior to the injured elder. Some reveal charming and winning personalities in public but in private (especially when dealing with elders) exhibit an immaturity, callousness, and cruelty that can be shocking. Sometimes the caregiver is a physically healthy but mentally impaired spouse while the victim, though physically handicapped, may be mentally healthy. As their individual conditions worsen, the outcome may be abuse.

Abusers often deny responsibility for injuries; instead, they will claim that bruises and broken bones resulted from a fall. However, the locations of these injuries preclude such explanations. Some justify ill treatment by accusing the abused elder of provoking abusive responses and thereby receiving what they deserve. Others express remorse after violence and promise not to do it again, only to repeat the abusive behavior—often with increased frequency and intensity. It has been observed that if the violence against, or neglect of, the elder had been perpetrated by a stranger, prosecution would follow, but when the abuse occurs at the hands of a relative, family members often support the abuser by remaining silent.

The reluctance of elders to report their abusive situations is based partially on loyalty to the family and partially on shame. The fear that the daughter or son may face trial and be sentenced to jail tugs at parental feelings of responsibility and loyalty. To be the reason for the incarceration of one's own child is, in the minds of some older adults, unthinkable; they prefer to suffer the indignities rather than betray family trust. Some are frightened at the prospect of being cut off from family and being compelled to live in a nursing home. Other elders are ashamed to admit that they have failed as parents in raising a child who abuses them. To confess to being abused by their offspring is to admit failure as a parent.

Still other elders feel that *somehow* they must be partially to blame for the treatment they receive. These older adults come out of a social and cultural environment in which punishment followed crime; they are being abused (punished), so they must have done something to deserve the treatment. When elder abuse involves maltreatment by a spouse, the fear of losing a home environment, difficult and cruel though it may be, is simply too threatening to one who is already insecure. Many prefer to remain quiet and endure their present situation.

WHAT CAN BE DONE?

How can we respond in instances where an elder is abused in the family, and what can be done to prevent such occurrences? Obviously the elder, the abuser, and the family are in need of professional counseling. Abusers need to understand the factors that trigger abusive behavior and learn that no person, no matter what age, sex, or social setting, is to be maltreated. They need to learn that there exists a no-tolerance attitude toward abuse and that further violations will result in punishment. The family must be helped to find new and better ways to solve problems and to resolve differences.

Battered elders need help in learning that they do not deserve abuse, no matter what the real or imagined behavior, and that there are resources available to help. To remain in an abusive situation is not an acceptable alternative. Victims of abuse must learn that they can adapt to a new environment, make new friends who will not violate their person or their rights, and that calling for help is an acceptable social response to abuse. Most important, society at large, through the media and instructional settings, must continue to expose abuse, inform the abused and their abusers of sources of help, strengthen a public no-tolerance attitude toward abuse, and encourage reporting wherever and whenever abuse occurs.

The rights and needs of caregivers also requires recognition. Most are not abusers and do not wish to abuse. It is not a simple or easy task to become responsible for a frail elder who brings into a familial relationship a distinct personality as well as a unique set of needs and demands. Accommodations are essential, but the needs and rights of caregivers must be addressed as well.

In 1985, The Andrus Volunteers at the University of Southern California published a booklet titled *Who Cares? Helpful Hints For Those Who Care for a Dependent Older Person.* Included was a "Caregivers' Bill of Rights" which read as follows:

Inasmuch as WE, THE CAREGIVERS, devote ourselves and our internal and external resources to the maintenance and support of a loved one, we declare that we have basic, inalienable rights. Furthermore, we recognize that we are not alone in our challenge to maintain a humane lifestyle for ourselves and our loved ones; therefore we pledge our support to all who struggle with balancing the responsibilities of daily living.

With this in mind we mandate the following rights:

The right to live our own lives and retain our dignity and sense of self.

The right to choose a plan of caring that accommodates our needs and the needs of those we care about.

The right to be recognized as a vital and stabilizing source within our families.

The right to be free of guilt, anguish, and doubt, knowing that the decisions we make are appropriate for our own well-being and that of our loved one.

The right to be ourselves enough to have confidence that we are doing the best that we are able.

With these rights, the disabled and frail elderly will be provided the highest and best care that we are capable of giving, and we may take pride in ourselves.

INSTITUTIONAL ABUSE

While many nursing homes provide excellent care for elders, others do not. Abuse in nursing homes is not always easy to detect. Periodic visits by state officials may be announced in advance providing the institution with the opportunity to "clean up" substandard conditions. Unannounced inspections often detect elder abuse, which may include:

- unsanitary conditions in kitchens, toilets, and rooms;

- neglect: elders left in their own urine or feces in beds that have not been changed in days;

- medical neglect: elders suffering from bedsores, some so grievous that they are infected with maggots;

- neglect of oral hygiene: mouth sores, poor fitting dentures, gum infections that receive no attention;

- overmedication: no attention is paid to medicines taken by the elder;

- sedation to keep elders quiet and uncomplaining;

- the use of psychotropic drugs that can turn elders "into drooling, incontinent zombies" (Spiegel 1991, p. 20);

- physical restraints that render the elder a prisoner, cause restraint burns, swellings, skins sores, and demoralized spirits;

- callous and brutal treatment ranging from verbal put-downs to slaps, pinching, pushes, shaking, to the bruising of the body and even breaking of bones;

- lack of stimulation in the environment: elders are left sitting in front of the television in states of semi-stupor;

- feeding problems: bed-bound elders have food placed where they cannot reach it, those who cannot feed themselves are ignored, others are brutally force fed;

- indifference to the psychological or familial problems that may be upsetting an elder;

- sexual abuse.

Although sexual abuse may not be common, the effects of the violation of another's body may be so serious and long-lasting that at least one reported case is worth noting. A one-hundred-pound woman suffering from Huntington's syndrome was allegedly raped by a nursing home aide as she was taken to have a shower (Sands 1990). She was provided with counseling by a therapist skilled in rape treatment. Nevertheless, the consequences of the violence perpetrated on her body simply did not go away, nor did the fact that her ailment, which reduced her to child-like dependency, erase the effects. Her feelings of security in the nursing home were affected. She was deprived of autonomy and control. Her "inner and most private space" was invaded by an assailant who used power and authority to violate her (Hartman and Burgess 1986, p. 2009). No small matter! Unfortunately, she is not alone.

Where do such cruel and uncaring people come from and why are they employed in the field of elder care? What do they symbolize in modern society? What prompts family members to place elders in nursing homes that fall so far below standards of quality care?

It is important to recognize that many who mistreat elders in nursing homes do not see themselves as cruel or uncaring. Indeed, they may protest that they are there because they care! Some, when confronted with their actions, are ashamed and confused by what they discover in themselves. In their own minds, they are not, by nature, mean people. Then, what happens to them in residential settings where elders look to them for help and support in confronting the declining years of life? According to B. F. Skinner (1972), abuse occurs when "those who exert control are subject to little or no countercontrol." He continues:

> In the absence of effective countercontrol those in charge begin to change—from being merely careless to being callous or even cruel. In the end they almost necessarily behave in ways we call ethically wrong. They do not do so because they lack compassion, but because reciprocal action has been weak or absent. What they may have at first felt as compassion grows weak or vanishes altogether.
>
> The care of the chronically ill or the aged is subject to the same deterioration. Nursing homes and homes for the elderly are often supported by the state or by relatives who take little further interest in what happens in them. The ill or the aged cannot protest effectively, nor can they escape, and little or no countercontrol is therefore exerted. Under these conditions those in charge begin to act in ways we call ethically wrong. They do so not because they lack compassion but because there is no adequate countercontrol, and as their behavior deteriorates, nothing is left to be felt as compassion. (p. 286)

It must be remembered, too, that institutional workers "burn out." Large hospitals and nursing homes are corporations. Worker dissatisfaction can be related to routines, to overwork in short-staffed settings, to low pay, to dead-end jobs, and so forth. This results in a depressed, dysfunctional staff. Janice Wood Wetzel (1984) notes that "depressed nurses or social workers, for example, controlled by physicians and their institutions and lacking a sense of competence and worth, may in turn treat their patients in a controlling manner" (p. 170).

Elders are placed in these poorly run, low-quality nursing homes by family members who are overburdened with problems and who are seeking release from elder care that is beyond their capacities to handle. They may examine several nursing homes and try to find ones they can afford; they end up choosing what seems to be the best within their price range.

In-depth investigations are not conducted. Instead, they are given a surface tour. When they visit their loved ones they are told that restraints or sedatives are necessary because of uncontrollable behavior problems. Unless they are feisty persons, there is a tendency to accept what appear to be logical explanations that might be enhanced with medical jargon. Until they become angry enough over the treatment, demand change, and state "No one treats my father or mother this way," thereby threatening public exposure or legal response, the nursing home continues its patterned treatments. One of the best allies elders have is the media. When newspapers, magazines, and television programs report elder mistreatment in words and pictures, reforms begin. Government inspectors become active interventionists (usually accompanying their long overdue responses with sad tales about how busy they are), legislators become incensed (suddenly) and demand reforms, district attorney's offices threaten legal action, letters to the editor express citizen outrage, and all at once society becomes concerned and involved with the welfare of its oldest members. If this is what it takes to reform and up-grade or to close down inferior nursing homes, then family members need to cultivate the media to render justice and to tap the human sense of decency.

Steps reflecting ethical concern must be taken within care-providing institutions. Every long-term care facility, every nursing home, every residential center for elders needs to have posted in a public place a client code of ethics regarding treatment. Every employee of the institution must be required to read, understand, and sign a statement of commitment to the principles enunciated in the code with the understanding that violation is grounds for dismissal. Upon admission, all residents must be told their rights and understand that there will be no toleration of abuse of any kind: verbal, psychological, physical, environmental, or spiritual. Each patient needs to know the ethical code by which the institution governs itself and understand the ways in which violations can be reported and dealt with.

An institutional ethical code might include the following:

We are committed to the health and well-being of all who live and work here. We will tolerate no use of language or gestures that denigrate another and this includes inappropriate or slurring references to racial, national, religious, sexual, physical or mental orientation, or status. We will treat one another with respect. We will not cause pain or physically abuse another in anyway. We will refrain from the use of restraints and medications to control our residents. We will provide medications for treatment of illness only as prescribed by the patient's physician or our resident physician. We will seek to lift spirits by positive reinforcement and encourage those who look to us for care and assistance to become actively involved—mentally and physically—so that they may make the most of their daily living. We will treat the frail, the very ill, and the dying with the respect and gentle care they deserve.

But codes are not enough. Potential nursing home workers must be screened to weed out persons with sadistic tendencies or with negative attitudes toward those of different race, religion, color, political, or sexual orientation, and so forth. Further, because mistreatment is often allied to stress, employee assistance programs need to be available through which stressed workers can find help in coping with feelings. Such programs act as internal safeguards against abuse and, when enhanced by regular governmental inspections, should serve to lessen abuse in long-term care facilities.

A statement of resident's rights could also be developed, which might read something like this:

As a resident you will be treated with respect and dignity and you are expected to treat others with respect and dignity. No resident or staff person will be subjected to verbal, physical, psychological, or financial abuse from another resident or from any staff person. Should violations occur, the abuser, whether resident or staff person, can face dismissal from the facility. You will be expected to respect the regulations we have developed for creating a healthy and homelike environment. All medications provided will be medically prescribed and will be given to better your health and to treat medically diagnosed illnesses. Resident are encouraged to seek ways to enhance their personal life and to participate in the opportunities provided by this residence to facilitate life enrichment.

As in the family setting, caregiver rights in the nursing home environment need recognition, too. Nursing home caregivers might come up with their own "Caregivers' Bill of Rights," which could read something like this:

Inasmuch as we, the nursing home caregivers, devote our time and energy to maintain and help the frail and dependent elders under our care, we declare that we have basic, inalienable rights. Furthermore, we recognize that we are not alone in our efforts to maintain a humane and dignified lifestyle both for ourselves and for the elders in our care; therefore, we pledge our support to all who struggle with balancing the responsibilities of daily work and daily living. With this in mind, we mandate the following rights:

- The right to live our own lives and retain our dignity and sense of self.

- The right to be involved in a plan of caring that recognizes and accommodates our needs as well as the needs of those we care about and serve.

- The right to be recognized as a vital and stabilizing source within our institutions.

- The right to work in a supportive environment that helps us to be free of guilt, anguish, and doubt, with the assurance that our services are appropriate for our own feelings of dignity and well-being as well as for the dignity and well-being of the elders we serve.

- The right to be ourselves enough to have confidence that we are doing the best that we are able.

With these rights, the disabled and frail elders whom we serve will be provided the highest and best care that we are capable of giving and we may take pride in ourselves and in our work.

BENIGN ABUSE

A more subtle form of abuse is practiced by families that abandon elder parents and relatives in nursing homes and retirement centers. Weeks and even months pass without any communication between the elder and the family. When the elder generates contact by letters or cards, they are ignored and left unanswered. If the effort to communicate is made by telephone, conversations are cut short and the elder is made to feel like an intruder.

The feelings of being discarded are enhanced when other members of the nursing home or center receive regular visits, letters, and phone calls from family members. Neglected elders may seek to preserve a falsified sense of family pride through lies that explain how busy their family members are. On the other hand, the elders may become angry and seek to punish their families through deleting names from wills (if there is any property to give). More often than not, these elders exist in lonely longing and psychic pain.

In institutional settings, where individuals are isolated and neglected by their families, volunteer visitors can help the isolated elder feel important. Sometimes, lonely elders find consolation and support in meeting and talking with others who have had similar experiences. Although, as Max Rosenbaum (1976) has pointed out, "every form of human activity is believed to be the source of some form of catharsis" (p. 6), such encounters should not be labeled "group therapy."

> Many people assume that when three or more individuals meet and talk about problems some type of group therapy is occurring. This is false. While in the broadest sense a certain kind of therapy is taking place, it is generally unplanned and may more accurately be described as nontherapeutic group interaction. It is what may happen when friends or acquaintances unload their problems to one another in a neighborhood bar or at a dinner party. (p. 2)

Through such encounters, isolated elders may discover that they are not alone, that others have similar experiences, and that through sharing, some of the damaged feelings may be partially repaired. Indeed, in some institutions several individuals meet regularly to chat and associate on an informal basis. When such meetings become the basis of friendships, those family members who regularly visit residents often extend their embrace to include the group, again alleviating feelings of isolation.

Institutional social workers often form groups to help isolated persons relate to others. Here the aim may be both social and therapeutic by providing settings where elders may air their feelings in the presence of a professional facilitator. Once again, isolated elders may discover that they are not alone, that others grapple with similar feelings. What is equally important is that out of such discussions come ways of coping with isolation and bonding with other elders.

On festive occasions, such as Christmas, various groups may visit nursing homes to sing carols, bring gifts, and talk with patients. Visits by children's groups are often most welcome inasmuch as children appear to be less inhibited in talking with elders and more affectionate with physical responses such as hugs and kisses. These are indeed noble and heart-warming endeavors, but the tendency is for elders to be ignored during the rest of the year. What is far more important are the regular visits by caring volunteers where patterns of recognition of individual elders are generated, helping to dispel feelings of being social discards without identity.

THE FUTURE

The elder boom is in its initial stages. The number of people over age seventy-five will continue to grow. At the same time, the number of women now entering the marketplace, many of whom will probably continue to be the main caregivers, shows no sign of decreasing; it is not impossible that their time, energy, and willingness to care for their aged parents or parents-in-law will diminish. The trend toward smaller families means that there will be fewer offspring available to share the responsibilities of elder-care. Economic fluctuations and the ever-increasing costs of medical care will continue to place financial strains on both the elderly and their families thereby contributing to the potential deterioration of family relationships. At present it is estimated that one out of every two first marriages ends in divorce, which results in increasing social strains on family relationships. Unless dramatic changes in medical care are made (including a national health insurance program in the United States) and unless efforts are made to alleviate the mounting stress manifested in family relationships, the future of present baby-boomers—those who will produce a crest in the number of elders in the years ahead—looks extremely bleak.

On the other hand, awareness of the fact that present problems cast shadows ahead, presents a challenge. Changes can be made. We are only beginning to deal with the social, economic, health, and family problems engendered by the new longevity. The ways in which we confront these challenges today will determine, in large part, the pattern of the future. Therefore, within the bleakness mentioned above, there are reasons for hope.

In the first place, more attention is being given to the causes of elder abuse, to the rescuing of abuse victims and to the rehabilitation of both the abusers and the abused. More and better information about elder abuse must be disseminated and more persons trained to recognize and deal with it. In view of the most recent studies, this training must include awareness of spousal abuse (particularly abuse of male spouses) among the elderly. It is imperative that the detection and reporting of elder abuse be enhanced. Such efforts require the mobilization and cooperation of public and private sectors to help victims. The community as a whole and special groups within the community—including social service agencies, churches, schools, and families—must, through workshops and educational efforts, engage in creating moral and ethical awareness geared toward diminishing and outlawing any form of abuse, whether directed at children, spouses, or elders.

Together with an emphasis on developing healthful family patterns, regulations governing retirement centers and nursing homes must be made and enforced. Provision must be made for financial and medical care of the abused elders, for dealing with alienated families, and for the rehabilitation of abusers. It is important to remember that efforts to rescue abused elders by nonprofessionals should be avoided. Social workers claim that interventions by untrained persons tend to create more problems than they solve.

It is also important that the polyglot nature of our developing society be recognized. Now, as never before in history, communities include families whose racial, cultural, and social mores may embrace customs that differ from traditional Western patterns. Many of these people are in transition and generational tensions develop within families. Those who deal with such groups must have knowledge of the language(s) and lifestyle(s) of these special groups. Social work departments in large multi-ethnic cities usually include trained workers with differing racial and cultural backgrounds who have the knowledge necessary for understanding familial patterns of special groups and the skills required to familiarize such groups with standard, accepted patterns.

Legislation must be supportive of and provide for the integration of intervention and protective services. Because elder abuse tends to involve repetitive abusive behavior, it is imperative that procedures be initiated for the immediate removal of the elder from a threatening situation. Then, not only must the abuser be required to undergo treatment, but therapy for the entire family is usually necessary. Should the abuser remain noncompliant, then provisions must be readily available for long-term protection of the victim. Such steps can be unnerving to victims, who will require assistance in modifying attitudes so that, out of respect for the self, they will recognize the importance of refusing to return to or remain in an abusive environment.

These important and necessary steps for the protection of elders will not come without a price. But ethical concern for the well-being of citizens, and in this case particularly older citizens, demands that changes be initiated and developed. Only then will it be possible to reduce and, we would hope, eliminate elder abuse.

REFERENCES

Andrus Volunteers. 1985. *Who Cares? Helpful Hints for Those Who Care for a Dependent Older Person at Home.* Los Angeles: University of Southern California Andrus Center.

Block, Marilyn R., and Jan D. Sinnot. 1979. *The Battered Elder Syndrome: An Exploratory Study.* Baltimore: University of Maryland Center on Aging.

Connelly, Michael. 1990. "Elderly Victim of Lincoln S&L Loss Takes Own Life," *The Los Angeles Times,* November 29.

Fulmer, T. T., and T. A. O'Malley. 1987. *Inadequate Care of the Elderly.* New York: Springer Publishing.

Fromm, Erich. 1973. *The Anatomy of Human Destructiveness.* New York: Holt, Rinehart and Winston.

Giordano, N. H., and J. A. Giordano. 1984. "Elder Abuse: A Review of the Literature," *Social Work* 29, pp. 223–26.

Goldstein, Jeffrey H. 1986. *Aggression and Crimes of Violence.* New York: Oxford University Press.

Hartman, Carol R., and Ann W. Burgess. 1986. "Sexual Trauma," in *Clinical Nursing,* June N. Thompson, Gertrude K. McFarland, Jane E. Hirsch, Susan M. Tucker, and Arden C. Bowers, eds. Princeton, N.J.: The C. V. Mosby Company, pp. 2009–16.

Jain, Kelly. 1990. "Project Counters Exploitation of Elderly," *The Los Angeles Times,* November 30.

Katz, Katheryn. 1980. "Elder Abuse," *Journal of Family Law,* June, pp. 695–722.

Lorenz, Konrad. 1966. *On Aggression.* New York: Harcourt Brace Jovanovich.

Mair, George. 1980. " 'Granny Bashing' Looms as Major Family Problem," *The Los Angeles Times,* November 7.

Neuman, Gerard G., ed. 1987. *Origins of Human Aggression.* New York: Human Sciences Press.

O'Malley, T. A., D. E. Everitt, H. C. O'Malley, and E. W. Campon. 1983. "Identifying and Preventing Family-Mediated Abuse and Neglect of Elderly Persons," *Annals of Internal Medicine* 98, pp. 998–1005.

Pillemer, K. A., and R. S. Wolf. 1986. *Elder Abuse: Conflict in the Family.* Massachusetts: Auburn House.

Pillemer, Karl, and David Finkelhor. 1988. "The Prevalence of Elder Abuse: A Random Sample Survey," *The Gerontologist* 28, no. 1, February, pp. 51–57.

Quinn, M. J., and S. K. Tomita. 1986. *Elder Abuse and Neglect.* New York: Springer Publishing.

Rosenbaum, Max. 1976. "Group Psychotherapy," in Max Rosenbaum and Alvin Snadowsky, eds., *The Intensive Group Experience.* New York: The Free Press, pp. 1–49.

Sands, Shannon. 1990. "Nursing Home Resident Says She Was Raped," *The Los Angeles Times,* August 17.

Seymour, E., ed. 1978. *Psychosocial Needs of the Aged: A Health Care Perspective.* Los Angeles: University of Southern California Press.

Skinner, B. F. 1972. "Compassion and Ethics in the Care of the Retardate," in *B. F. Skinner: Cumulative Record.* New York: Meredith Corporation, pp. 283–91.

Spiegel, Claire. 1991. "Restraints, Drugging, Rife in Nursing Homes," *The Los Angeles Times,* March 25.

Star, Barbara. 1983. *Helping the Abuser.* New York: Family Service Association.

Steinmetz, Suzanne K. 1988. *Duty Bound: Elder Abuse and Family Care.* Newbury Park, Calif.: Sage Publications.

Storr, Anthony. 1986. *Human Aggression.* New York: Atheneum.

Wetzel, Janice Wood. 1984. *Clinical Handbook of Depression.* New York: Gardner Press.

8

Geroethics and Religion

"Religion is one of the most important of the many ways in which Americans 'get involved' in the life of their community and society."

—Bellah et al., *Habits of the Heart,* p. 219

From time to time throughout this book, there have been references to the relationship of belief systems to aging and to the lives of elders. Here the emphasis will be on the Western religious tradition simply because it plays the largest role in the Western world.

Religion in Western civilization has drawn its inspiration primarily from the Bible, in which the deity is referred to in both transcendent and imminent terms. The transcendent God is distant, powerful, in control, and Lord and King of his creation. The imminent God is a close, warm, nurturing, and protective Father figure. During fear of cataclysmic storms, earthquakes, floods, or other natural disasters, appeal is made to the transcendent God to control nature and to deliver his followers. When personal tragedies occur or when individuals feel helpless and insecure, prayers go out to the immanent Father God to reveal caring and to provide succor. The moving hymn "Abide with Me" touches on the theme of the deity as caregiver: "When other helpers fail and comforts flee, O Thou, who failest not, abide with me," and asks that "In life, in death, O Lord, abide with me." It is to the transcendent-immanent god-image that believing humans turn during life's crises.

Whether or not comfort and release is provided, the believer trusts that God is in charge. If the hurricane misses the prayer's home, then the prayer was answered, despite the fact that other homes occupied, perhaps by other prayerful people, were destroyed. If human help arrives to bring changes in the life of the troubled person, it is assumed that God answered the prayer and sent that succor. If aid fails to materialize, God has said no and believers can blame themselves for the refusal. God never fails, humans do. Obviously, religion can furnish either toxic or nourishing attitudes toward the self and toward life.

THE TOXIC AND THE NOURISHING

Where religion serves to integrate the personality and links the individual to a life philosophy or a life work that provides meaning, it can be said to be nourishing. Where religion provokes fear and insecurity and self-blame, it can be said to be toxic. Take the case of my father who was, throughout his life, a devout Roman Catholic. His final years were marked with concern for the after-life. He had been raised to believe in the existence of hell, purgatory, and heaven and that each person would, in the after-life, end up in one of those places. His life had not been easy, and in the minds of some he could have been said to have experienced something of a personal hell-on-earth. During his last years, he attended Roman Catholic services regularly, prayed often, said his rosary, and paid for masses to be said in his name after his death. These were not comfortable or comforting notions. He was insecure and could not trust his God to understand. Perhaps he was unsure about the legends of the divine Mary, the compassionate mother figure, who could help the rejected into heaven by an alternative route. Perhaps my father found some comfort in the hope that somehow justice would be meted out in the hereafter. What was most obvious was his insecurity. To the outside observer, his faith system was more toxic than nourishing. For him, the nourishing dimensions were in the belief that there would be another and perhaps a better life beyond this one.

There are other toxic potentials in religion: among them the vulnerability of lonely and isolated elders to the wiles of persuasive and unethical clergy who employ Bible quotations (usually lifted out of context) and the language of guilt and obligation to encourage elders to contribute to a variety of programs and projects. An elderly woman, featured on a major television talk show, said that she had contributed half a million dollars to a Christian cult whose minister quoted scripture and sought to isolate both her and her money from her family. She was rescued and deprogrammed by her daughters who, when they had difficulty in communicating with her, recognized that she was the victim of a religious scam.

One need only listen to television evangelists to become aware of the pressure put on shut-ins and others who fill part of their lonely days by listening to religious programs, seeking comfort from the God they had been raised to trust. These evangelists stress over and over again that "giving to God" (by which they mean contributing to their particular programs) would bring blessings. They promise (some seem almost to guarantee) the contributor everything from monetary rewards or physical benefits in this life to entry into heaven in the next. Once the donation is made, the mail from the evangelist increases. Letters that appear to be personally addressed to the donor are, of course, computer produced and composed by skilled sales persons who know which emotional buttons to push to produce a response. In all such instances, the religion is toxic and ultimately has toxic effects on the person. But toxic religious practice is not limited to these unethical clergy.

After the death of her husband, who had been a successful business man, a seventy-year-old woman sold the family home for well over a million dollars in excess of what it had cost. She then moved into a comfortable condominium in a retirement community where she felt secure in the knowledge that she was well provided for. She was soon approached by the president of her husband's college—a small but respectable religious institution—and was urged to commit close to a million dollars to establish a chair in her husband's name. The approach was cordial and at a high level but loaded with the religious "oughts" and "shoulds" destined to produce guilt if she failed to comply. She was troubled and somewhat confused by the pressure, but wise enough to stall. She said she needed time to get her affairs in order. As she weighed the urgings by the college against her needs for the future, she made a decision guided by legal counsel.

Now, of course, not all religion can be classified as toxic. Many denominations sponsor retirement and nursing homes for the elderly where they are made to feel important and where their faith contributed to their sense of personal meaning. They live in a protected environment in which the positive elements of Judaism or Christianity are demonstrated. The community of faith helps to regenerate the personality as these elders begin to feel alienation from the larger world. Here the identity is not so much in terms of work nor even of family, but as members of a caring group uniquely attached to the God of the faith system. The caring aspects of the deity are manifested in the caring responses of the retirement community.

In some local churches, one or more members of the clergy team and special committees are set up to minister specifically to the needs of elders. Housebound elders are visited, transported to and from institutional activities, prayed over and prayed with, and made to feel important and significant. In some instances, the caring outreach embraces the entire family and continues to be effective after the death of the elder. Such humanistic outreach cannot be faulted and can only be evaluated as nourishing.

Hospital and nursing home chaplains play important roles. In most instances, these persons have received special training that equips them to deal with elderly patients. They become the elders' friends and confidants. The clergy may act as intermediaries when tensions arise between elders and their families. Chaplains may respond to the needs of the elderly in ways that institutional workers cannot. What may be most important is their presence and their counsel when an elder is dying and the family is in shock and grieving (Sweetser 1985, pp. 136ff).

In the epigram to this chapter, Robert N. Bellah and his co-writers comment on the important role of religion in providing a means for social involvement. The ideal is not always realized by elders. Some religious organizations tend to segregate them within an array of special groups for young people, for young married couples, and for the elderly. Like so many other institutions, hospitals and nursing homes have accepted the notion that elders prefer to talk among themselves and have little or nothing to share with younger age-groups. In many religious communities elders are simply there—not truly involved, not really known, but just there with all their unexplored potential.

Elder wisdom, which in the past was honored and appreciated in religious settings, tends to be ignored; elders are seen and acknowledged but are unused.

AGE AND RELIGION

Despite the claims, there is no evidence that as persons get older they become more religious. It was so in my father's case, but it is not so in the lives of other elders. There is also no way to determine the increase or decrease in elders' degree of participation in religion; such involvement can be measured on different scales. Is the participation to be evaluated in terms of involvement in church programs, in terms of attendance, in terms of an increase in personal devotional activities, in terms of financial support, in terms of the number of radio or television programs listened to or watched, or in terms of fidelity to a given belief system (Atchley 1972, pp. 279ff)?

How is the life of an elder who lives a good, decent, ethical existence to be evaluated? Some years ago, I subjected a number of Christian congregations to a hypothetical situation:

> Here is a man who likes to attend congregational meetings. He approves of their community services program that seeks to help the elderly, the youth, young married couples, parents in the sandwich generation, and so on. He enjoys the clergy and the sermons, the people and their attitude. He is a good, decent human being who likes what they are about and who supports their efforts with healthy financial giving. In spite of the fact that he does not accept their theology (which I always defined in terms of that of the particular denomination), he would like to become a member of the church. Would they accept him?

The discussions that followed were fascinating and the voting on whether to admit this fictional person usually revealed the diversity of belief about what constituted religion in the minds of the members of the congregation. Indeed, some became so involved that I received phone calls for more than a week afterward from persons who wanted to change their vote either pro or con. I was not particularly interested in how the vote turned out, but in the process by which different persons in a given church approached their religion. The issue is still pertinent. If an elder becomes more involved in social and religious programs that reach out to the less fortunate persons in the community, is that person becoming more religious or simply more socially aware, and is there a difference? Or does the person simply have more time since retirement to be involved in these important human efforts? Is the belief system really that important? Many elders have moved away from concepts they embraced as children, but keep an affiliation with the church of their childhood; are they more or less religious? Such questions indicate the difficulty in attempting to use statistical data or to try to force upon elders the theory that they become either more or less religious as they age. Some studies focus on small groups of elders within a given religious community and tell us only what has occurred in the lives of members of that group. Other studies focus on value changes and adjustment outside of a purely faith context. The studies do not provide us with information that can be applied in general to elders.

This same ambivalence appears in Barbara Myerhoff's study (1979) of the community of elderly Jews living in Venice, California. Her book, *Number our Days,* is laced through with references to traditional Judaism, but the religious character of the community ranges from Humanism to a kind of Orthodoxy. I suspect that her account, written from a sociological standpoint, reflects the real complexion of elders and religion.

In a study of elders in San Francisco, Clark and Anderson (1967) noted that church attendance was more frequent among mentally ill elders than among the mentally healthy. This suggested that mentally ill elders tended to be anxious and fearful and found emotional support in religion. Clark and Anderson also suggested that the mentally ill could become obsessed with religion, just as they could become obsessed with almost anything else. These elders had a need to know about immortality and about what happens after death. These individuals differed from the control group for whom religion was not an obsession but had social value (pp. 328–45). As Atchley comments, "Of course, this finding does not mean that most older people who attend church are mentally ill; it simply means that the *proportion* who regularly attend church was significantly higher among mentally ill older people than among other older people in the sample studied by Clark and Anderson" (p. 281). He adds, "Clark and Anderson's findings may also be confounded by the fact that their sample came from California, where people of all ages attend church less frequently than in other regions of the United States" (p. 281). Atchley notes:

> Contrary to popular belief, interest and participation in religious activities does not appear to protect people from loneliness or fear of death, nor do lonely people tend to turn to religion. . . . Only the most conservative of religious people show serenity and a decreasing fear of death. . . . On other personal dimensions, such as self-esteem, identity, attitudes, values, beliefs, and norms, religion appears to increase in importance with age. Again, however, we do not know if this increase is a change with age or simply an intergenerational difference. (p. 283)

More than twenty-five years ago, I teamed up with Professor Robert Leslie of the Pacific School of Religion in Berkeley, California, to distribute a questionnaire among senior couples in a large Methodist church in the area. We were attempting to determine the use of a daily devotional guide that had been given to each couple by the church. We separated husbands and wives, so that they were not able to collaborate on answers. The results were interesting because of the differences in responses. Quite often, one spouse would write that the couple used the guide every day, while the other would indicate that they did not engage in daily devotions or that they seldom looked at the guide. We became dubious about the response that the church usually released when it reported on the use of the devotional pamphlet.

Shortly afterward, I developed a set of questions that I used in a number of Presbyterian, Methodist, and Congregational churches on the West Coast in which I queried religious experience and "answers to prayer." My present memory of the results was that many church-going elders (those over sixty-five) appeared to have had deep and moving religious experiences in which they felt a personal contact with the deity, while the youth described their religious experiences in terms of aesthetic responses to nature such as sunsets at a youth camp, for example. The same was true of responses to prayer: senior church members believed they were in deep personal communication with the deity, while the youth were not so sure. One young woman (a minister's daughter) commented: "Prayer is like talking into the telephone without being sure anyone is on the other end." Inasmuch as I have long since discarded the hundreds of sheets of paper that recorded the responses and I am relying on memory, the results I report have no real statistical value. Then, too, those same young people are now well into middle age and may have had different experiences that would affect their responses, while the elders who responded would be, for the most part, dead. The vibrancy of some of our conservative churches with huge congregations numbering in the thousands (in California!) suggests that there are many persons of all ages seeking and perhaps finding meaning in religion. Perhaps it is time for new surveys!

There can be little question that for many lonely and isolated persons, the outreach of the synagogue and church are important and life-affirming, nor can the importance of a personal belief system be underestimated. To believe that there is a God who cares and who can be accepted as a friend and comforter is a source of strength for many elders.

REFERENCES

Achenbaum, W. Andrew. 1985. "Religion in the Lives of the Elderly," in Gari Lesnoff-Caravaglia, ed., *Values, Ethics and Aging.* New York: Human Sciences Press, Inc., pp. 98–116.
Atchley, Robert C. 1972. *The Social Forces in Later Life.* Belmont, Calif.: Wadsworth Publishing Company, Inc.

Bellah, Robert N., et al. 1985. *Habits of the Heart.* New York: Harper and Row.

Clark, Margaret, and Barbara Anderson. 1967. *Culture and Aging.* Springfield, Ill.: Charles C. Thomas.

Larue, Gerald A. 1979. "Biblical Mythology and Aging," *Gerontology in Higher Education.* Wadsworth, pp. 81–90.

————. 1981. "Religion and the Aged," in Irene Mortenson Burnside, ed., *Nursing and the Aged.* New York: McGraw-Hill Book Company (2nd edition) pp. 642–50.

————. 1985. "Historical Perspectives on the Role of the Elderly: The Most Ancient Evidence," in Gari Lesnoff-Caravaglia, ed., *Values, Ethics and Aging.* New York: Human Sciences Press, pp. 41–55.

Markides, Kyriakos S. 1987. "Religion," *The Encyclopedia of Aging.* New York: Springer Publishing Company, pp. 559–61.

Moberg, David O. 1967. "Some Findings and Insight from My Research on Religion and Aging," in *Religion and Aging.* Los Angeles: University of Southern California, pp. 27–45.

Myerhoff, Barbara. 1979. *Number our Days.* New York: E. P. Dutton.

Palmore, Erdman. 1987. "Religious Organizations," *The Encyclopedia of Aging.* New York: Springer Publishing Company, pp. 561–63.

Sweetser, Carleton J. 1985. "Hospital Clergy and the Elderly Patient," in Gari Lesnoff-Caravaglia, ed., *Values, Ethics and Aging.* New York: Human Sciences Press, pp. 136–57.

Swenson, Wendell M. 1967. "Approaches to the Study of Religion and Aging," in *Religion and Aging.* Los Angeles: University of Southern California, pp. 59–81.

9

Elders and the Work Ethic

"In a general 'socio-economic' sense 'work' includes all activities presumed to contribute to a society's existence and survival, that is, activities involved in the production and distribution of all life-sustaining and life-enhancing goods and services, as well as ritualistic activities. Participation in 'work' at appropriate stages during the life cycle is the usual basis for an individual's claim to a share in his society's manifold resources."

—Gil, *Unravelling Social Policy*, p. 66

This brief discussion of the work ethic will serve as an introduction to the larger treatment of "The Search for Meaning" (see chapter 10). The link is rather obvious, because for many elders it is important to be or to feel useful and feeling useful is often linked to work, to doing something that results in a product or payment or recognition. In some societies, the ability to contribute to the welfare of the group is directly linked to survival.

In migratory and hunting and gathering societies, the worth of an individual may be evaluated by the actual contribution made to the group. For example, A. R. Holmberg studied the Siriono of Bolivia and offers the following observation:

Since status is determined largely by immediate utility to the group, the inability of the aged to compete with the younger members of the society places them somewhat in the category of excess baggage. Having outlived their usefulness they are relegated to a position of obscurity. Actually the aged are quite a burden. They eat but are unable to hunt, fish, or collect food; they sometimes hoard a young spouse, but are unable to beget children; they move at a snail's pace and hinder the mobility of the group. . . . When a person becomes too ill or infirm to follow the fortunes of the band, he is abandoned to shift for himself. (Quoted in Watson and Maxwell 1977, p. 30)

The pattern is like that of certain Kurdish tribes. When they move their flocks from the plains to the mountains in the spring of the year, elders who are too feeble to cross swollen streams are left behind. Among some Eskimo, a feeble elder who is no longer able to contribute to family needs will go out in the arctic night and sit in the cold until he or she freezes to death. Utility is the key factor in these cultures. Only contribution to group welfare justifies or guarantees existence.

In the eyes of many persons in our society, people are what they do. After introductions, the first question is often "What do you do?" not "Who are you?" which could prompt a completely different answer. We are so conditioned that the response to either question is usually the same: "I am a policeman," "I am a teacher," or "I am *just* a housewife" (reflecting the demeaning of status for someone who lacks a professional, money producing label!) or even worse, "I'm retired" (useless?). We are recognized as persons, as important human beings, by what we do, by what we produce, not by the qualities we possess.

One might respond to the second question by saying "I am a loyal, trustworthy person actively involved in trying to make this world a better place in which to live for myself and for others." Does that sound too pompous, too evasive? Are some of the highest values that identify a person worthy of exposition and of relating to the self? These are values that can be part of the life of the policeman, the teacher, the housewife, the house*husband,* the retiree, or of any individual. Identification by and through work is a key factor in the work ethic, which suggests that individual worth is to be measured by the work one does.

The work ethic is not new. It did not suddenly appear with the industrial revolution as some have suggested. It has been with us for millennia and it is to be found in some of our oldest literature. For example, meaning and work are linked in the legend of King Gilgamesh of Uruk, the Sumerian ruler whose wondrous legend influenced Babylonian, Assyrian, Hittite, Canaanite, and Hebrew thought (including the story of the biblical flood). Although we shall meet Gilgamesh again in the discussion on longevity, his story is worth telling in some detail here.

According to an ancient Sumerian king-list, Gilgamesh ruled the city of Uruk in the third millennium B.C.E. Posthumously, he attained legendary status and was said to have been the offspring of a human male and a goddess; consequently, Gilgamesh was bigger, stronger, and more powerful than other humans. He exercised his semi-divine strength and regal status without regard for his people, possessing virgins prior to their marriage and bullying the men.

The people complained to the gods and a companion named Enkidu was created. After a violent physical encounter, the two men became friends and now Gilgamesh diverted his anti-social energy and behavior into endeavors directed against territories beyond Uruk. Whereas formerly he had found personal meaning through maltreatment of his people, now, together with Enkidu, he sought identity as a hero by defeating mythical monsters. This value system failed when the two companions violated territory belonging to the gods and offended a goddess. The divine assembly met and decided that one of the two offenders should die. Enkidu was selected.

Enkidu did not die a meaning-filled, heroic death. He died miserably in Gilgamesh's arms. At first, Gilgamesh refused to acknowledge his companion's death. For seven days and nights he held Enkidu in his arms until a maggot dropped from the dead man's nostrils and Gilgamesh suddenly became aware of his own mortality: "When I die, will I not be just like Enkidu?" he asked.

Never doubting the validity of his belief in a way of life that provided meaning by way of strength and authority, Gilgamesh determined to defeat death. He decided to visit his ancestor Utnapishtim, who had been awarded immortality by the gods because it was he who had preserved specimens of human and animal life on board his ship during the flood (Utnapishtim was the Sumerian predecessor of the biblical Noah). As he began his new venture, Gilgamesh paused for refreshment at an ale-house where the barmaid commented on the folly of his quest and suggested a different response to life:

> Gilgamesh, where are running?
> You won't find the immortal life you are seeking.
> When the gods created humankind
> They ordained death for humans
> And retained immortality for themselves.
> So Gilgamesh, let your belly be full.
> Be merry every day and night.
> Make each day a day of joy.

Dance, play by day and night.
Wear fresh clothes.
Let your head be anointed and your body bathed in water.
Cherish the child who grasps your hand.
Let your wife rejoice in your arms
For this is the destiny of humankind. . . .

The king dismissed her wisdom. The idea that meaning in life was based on the recognition that life is limited and that companionship, love, and enjoyment in living are to be sought rather than the manifestation of power did not coincide with Gilgamesh's beliefs.

He continued his journey, finally meeting up with Utnapishtim only to learn that the immortality granted to his ancestor was a special reward; it was not available to Gilgamesh. As a consolation, Utnapishtim told him about a magical root that grew beneath the sea, which when eaten would, by virtue of its rejuvenating power, make "the old man become as the young man." Gilgamesh acquired the root, but decided to delay eating it until he was older. As he washed away the sea water in a fresh water pool, a snake devoured the root, giving rise to an ancient explanation (which is noted in chapter 11 on "Longevity") as to why the snake sheds its skin and renews itself while humans are destined to wrinkle and age.

Gilgamesh had no choice but to return to his people. He had learned that meaning in life was not to be found in the ruthless exercise of power without regard for the rights of others, nor was it to be found in the heroic deeds through which he had hoped to achieve immortal stature. The simple day-by-day joy in living suggested by the barmaid was inadequate for him and, as he discovered, neither rejuvenation nor immortality were available. What could he do? How could he discover meaning, purpose, and significance for his life? To achieve his goal, Gilgamesh developed the work ethic. He became a great ruler, the defender of the citizens of Uruk, and the builder of the city's protective walls. His meaning, his destiny, was to be found in the fulfillment of his role as king, i.e., in the work ethic, not in pursuing adventures elsewhere.

There was a message to be found in the account of Gilgamesh's adventures. Those who read and heard his story learned that if the search for the meaning of life through power and glory pursued by a semi-divine king had failed for this superman, such searches would surely not prevail for the ordinary person. The real answer to life, living, and the pursuit of meaning or happiness was to be found in work.

Gilgamesh busied himself with kingly duties. He refurbished the temples of Anu, the patron god of Uruk, to bring divine blessings to the city, and of Ishtar, the goddess of fertility and love, to promote amicable relations and fecundity of crops, herds, and families. The true meaning of his life came through work as Gilgamesh accepted the responsibilities of his position as ruler. In the same way, meaning would come to anyone who fulfilled his or her personal work responsibilities. In other words, work, responsibly executed, was the key to finding purpose and identity in life.

The biblical creation epic echoes the same doctrine. Adam and Eve were expelled from the garden of Eden because they ate fruit from the tree of moral/ethical knowledge. This act of disobedience raised them to a level of moral awareness exceeding that of their animal companions, but it failed to give them the potential for immortality, which, in the story, was associated with the tree of life. Adam and Eve were quickly expelled from paradise before they could eat of the tree of immortality, thus they were condemned to work to survive. They were told:

> The ground is cursed because of you, through work you shall derive your food from it all the days of your life. It will produce thorns and thistles for you even as you consume its field plants. You will get your bread by the sweat of your brow until you return to the ground. (Gen. 2:17-19)

In view of this notion of a divine destiny that ordains the need to work, it is not surprising to find that idleness is denigrated in the Bible (Prov. 19:15, 31:27; 2 Thess. 3:8).

Much later, Qoheleth, the teacher in Ecclesiastes, advised his pupils that pleasure (wine, women, and song), wealth and possessions, or even work itself would not give meaning to the meaninglessness of life. Nevertheless, because humans were trapped in a system of meaningless existence, all that was left was to accept the reality. The wisdom was expressed in the saying: "There is nothing better for a man than that he should eat and drink and find pleasure in his work" (Eccles. 2:24). Qoheleth recognized that, for humans, some choices were better than others. Like the barmaid, he advised his listeners to eat bread and drink wine with a merry spirit, to wear white garments, and to enjoy life with their wives, but Qoheleth adds, "Whatever your hand finds to do, do it with your might" (Eccles. 9:7-10). He recognized the importance of work for survival.

The work ethic is, therefore, our human heritage, developed by our ancestors as a principle of group survival, set forth in legendary and religious frameworks, and passed on through the ages to the present. Because of this ethic, in the eyes of many, we are what we do. We are important to the degree that our work contributes to the well-being of the group. It is assumed that work produces wealth and one might assume that the worthiest workers are the best paid and accumulate the most wealth. But this is not necessarily so. Every so often we are reminded that sometimes the routine jobs, those we take for granted, can be very important for group survival. For example, a trash collectors' strike in a major city can result in garbage piling up on sidewalks, rat infestations, the spread of disease, and so forth. Perhaps those who are responsible for collecting trash need to be paid in proportion to the importance of the service they perform!

Does this emphasis on the importance of work place elders in a difficult position? When we can no longer work and contribute, are we to be abandoned like the elders in the tribal systems described above?

Our ancestors were conscious of the lurking dangers that could befall elders when they became feeble. They produced laws, teachings, and principles—which they declared came from the mouths of their deities—that called for the honoring of parents and of elders. Once respect and care for elders became a cultural norm supported by divine law, it was believed that violations could offend the deity and bring punishment on the family or society that ignored the precept. The concept is found throughout the ancient Near East (Larue 1985) and in the teachings of Far Eastern philosophies and religion. The regulations reflect the insecurity of the aged and the steps influential elders took to safeguard their status and existence. They knew that guilt and fear could be very powerful motivators.

In societies where the aged are considered to be sources of wisdom, knowledge, or information, elders are held in respect. In the modern age this notion has undergone change. Data banks can provide instant recovery of information in quantities and detail far greater than that available from the memories of elder citizens. The wisdom and the insights of elders are often treated as obsolete, quaint, or to be politely listened to and endured when there is no escape. In view of these changing attitudes, it is not surprising that some elders experience feelings of insecurity when they retire and assume the status of nonproducers.

Of course, elders who are supported and cared for within a family setting may be in a somewhat different situation. As we shall see, their memories, stories, and anecdotes are accepted as important because they are part of family history. Their wisdom comes from experiences embedded within a familial context and therefore has meaning for the intimate group. Many elders have been encouraged to record their reminiscences and experiences for posterity, for the unborn offspring of the future. In such circumstances their life, their work, their retirement from productive society is converted into a new productivity that has special meaning for the family group.

We cope with nonproductivity in the aged in a number of ways. Wherever possible we keep them out of sight. Healthy retired elders retreat to Leisure World where they live together with other nonproducing elders. The social environment poses no threat. There every person is nonproductive (in a sense), living on the earnings and investments of the past. The elderly residents are free to putter at whatever interests them—golf, swimming, reading, writing, painting, and so forth. Frail, nonproductive elders go to nursing homes where they are looked after by a paid staff and visited by relatives and friends. Once again, they are kept out of sight and their uselessness is catered to in an environment where everything is done for them.

The mounting criticism of the costs of housing and care for the elderly can be unsettling. Recent events in history remind us how thin is the veneer of culture and civilization and how quickly it can be stripped away in times of crisis. In a period of worldwide economic depression, what protective safeguards would elders have? We like to believe that our Western societies have moved a long way from what happened in Nazi Germany and from the deceptive announcement that "work will make you free" that was proclaimed there. We recall that pre-Nazi Germany was a cultured, deeply religious nation committed to a Christian ethic that embraced honor and respect for elders. Overnight, so to speak, principles and ideals were abandoned and replaced with an ethic that stated that only through work was one entitled to freedom and support. The slogan "work will make you free" implied that those whom the Nazis determined were lesser human beings could survive only through their ability to work and serve the state. Feeble elders were not able to produce and could therefore be eliminated. How close are we to such a frightening immoral stance?

It is important to listen to the rhetoric of politics, of industry, and of bigotry to discern the faint rumblings of elder prejudice. Inflation pushes increasing numbers of elders toward poverty, where their welfare becomes the responsibility of government. These men and women believed their savings, their Social Security benefits, and their pension plans would guarantee them a decent, secure retirement. As the saved dollar shrinks in value, security is threatened. As the purchasing power of their fixed incomes diminishes, the quality of life is threatened. Some protection may be afforded through the impact of many elders on the marketplace, but in reality the elderly cannot count on the power of their dollars to guarantee protection. Like any minority group, they must know that it is only through the power to be heard and to affect legislation and the economy that their cries for help will be heeded.

The work ethic is here to stay. Perhaps the time has come to reevaluate our retirement policies, to heed the requests of those elders who love to work and who are capable of continuing to work. In some instances, perhaps jobs can be shared so that no excessive work load will fall on the shoulders of a single elder. But many older adults want to continue to feel productive. They do not thrive away from the work in which they are proficient. Some of our happiest elders are engaged in jobs that recognize their ability to perform without feeling stressed. Of course, some will not be able to work at the same pace as younger individuals, but they need not be employed where the two age groups are competing. Take the example of a sixty-nine-year-old male who loves sports. A sports arena has hired him, along with some younger men, to help individuals find their seats, to be part of the sports center staff. He is paid a minimum wage and he has the opportunity to watch the games. It is part-time work that he truly enjoys. Some have claimed that elders make excellent employees. They tend to be reliable, punctual, steady, trustworthy, and take fewer sick leaves. Of course, every elder will not be employable and some will not want to continue working, but for those who do, the doors of opportunity should remain open.

At the same time, society must find ways to accept and protect those elders who for personal, physical, or other reasons are no longer engaged in productive work. The work ethic has its place, but so does an ethic that respects the right to retire and seek from society the rewards of a lifetime of service.

REFERENCES

Gil, David G. 1976, 1981. *Unravelling Social Policy.* Cambridge, Mass.: Schenkman Publishing Co.

Larue, Gerald A. 1985. "Historical Perspectives on the Role of the Aging," in Gari Lesnoff-Caravaglia, *Values, Ethics and Aging.* New York: Human Sciences Press, Inc., pp. 41–55.

Watson, Wilbur, and Robert Maxwell. 1977. *Human Aging and Dying.* New York: St. Martin's Press.

10

Aging and the Search for Meaning

"If we hope to live not just from moment to moment but in true consciousness of our existence, then our greatest need and most difficult achievement is to find meaning in our lives."

—Bettelheim, *The Uses of Enchantment,* p. 3

Many individuals, perhaps most, tend to live their lives "from moment to moment" without asking about life's meaning. The issue may come to mind from time to time, but pondering about it can be put off. It is when one approaches the end of life that questions arise: "What is life all about?" or "What is the meaning of my life?" And the answers will vary.

Of course, meaning-filled living is always in process. Meaning lies in moments—in sacred or special moments that take on significance until, like a string of beads, they begin to form their own chain of identity and pattern. The sequence signifies growth and change and development. Meaning never "is" in the sense of being total or final, for to reach the point of completion would be to enter stasis or stagnation without growth or development. In such a state the ripening or continuing maturation of the life process would have reached a point of no growth, and without growth there is no development. The result would be the death of the spirit and, ultimately, of life itself. To believe or feel that existence has meaning requires reflection on what one's personal life means in particular. Let us examine some of the ways that individuals find meaning in life.

SELF-AWARENESS

Obviously, the organ of meaning is the brain. The decline and death of cognitive capacities robs the person of any awareness of or concern for meaning. For this very reason, visits to some nursing homes can be soul shaking experiences. So many of the inhabitants seem to have reached that point of no growth where life is not experienced, it just is. It can be questioned whether some of these elders who sit helplessly with glazed eyes or closed eyes, mouth agape, unable to communicate in any intelligible way, have any thoughts about meaning or purpose or destiny. They appear to have no capacity for abstract thought. There is no way of knowing what may be taking place in their minds—perhaps memories of things past, perhaps nothing at all.

Without the ability to reason, to evaluate, to make conscious choices, the individual is reduced to nonrational levels of response without the potential for appreciation of the notion of meaning. Such incapacitated people might provide meaning for caretakers who fulfill themselves through their ability to help others, but for the patient, when the ability to respond intellectually is forever lost, there can be no awareness of significance. Our discussion, therefore, will have two dimensions: first, meaning for the mentally aware; second, meaning for those whose cognitive abilities are reduced or gone.

RELIGION

Some claim to find life's meaning in a religious belief system. They accept the teachings of their particular group as authoritative or divinely revealed, and insofar as they live in accordance with the tenets of the faith system, they are fulfilling their life's meaning. A variety of options have developed within religions: one may belong to an orthodox or traditional group, to a liberal or reformed group, or to a body that claims for itself some new authoritative way of life.

For example, the eminent orthodox Jewish teacher Dr. Louis Finkelstein (1949, 1955), described orthodox Judaism as follows:

> Judaism is a way of life that endeavors to transform virtually every human action into a means of communion with God. Through this communion with God, the Jew is enabled to make his contribution to the establishment of the Kingdom of God and the brotherhood of men on earth. So far

as its adherents are concerned, Judaism seeks to extend the concept of right and wrong to every aspect of their behavior. Jewish rules of conduct apply not merely to worship, ceremonial, and justice between man and man, but also to such matters as philanthropy, personal friendships and kindnesses, intellectual pursuits, artistic creation, courtesy, the preservation of health, and the care of diet. (p. 1327)

Communion with God and the establishing of God's kingdom represent the purpose of life. Personal meaning is found through participation in that purpose. For the orthodox Jew, the teachings found in the Torah (the Jewish scriptures) and the Talmud (Jewish civil and religious law) provide guidance.

Conservative Jews tend to be more flexible. They view their faith as a living tradition subject to changes that must be in accord with the basic precepts of the Bible and the Talmud. Reform Jews are more prone to liberal interpretation of traditional canons and Humanistic Jews are secularists either ignoring or denying belief in the existence of a God. For this last group, finding meaning for life in Judaism expressed in orthodoxy has no relevance and represents a clinging to an outdated, chauvinistic faith system.

Exactly the same patterns can be found within Christianity which is based on the teachings of the Bible, in particular on the New Testament. Here, too, fulfilling the will of God and the establishment of the Kingdom of God are related to meaning for life; individual Christians find meaning in working toward the achievement of those purposes. Much emphasis is placed on the notion of "salvation," which guarantees the individual forgiveness of sin; identity with Jesus, the founder of the faith; and a place in the heaven of the afterworld. As in Judaism, the scriptures and the interpretations of sacred writings give guidances for ethical stances and behavior. Christianity also embraces a variety of faith expressions ranging from monastic life to vigorous evangelism, from staunch fundamentalism to a liberalism that is so involved in reinterpreting the Bible to fit modern secular life that it verges on Humanism. Multifaceted faith patterns can be extended to include Islam, Hinduism, Buddhism, and so forth. Each belief system presents a spectrum embracing literalists, dogmatists, and fundamentalists at one end and, at the other, religious secularists who for one reason or another cling to an identifying religious label while abandoning traditional requirements of the faith.

Insofar as religion links individuals to a community of faith that asserts and reasserts their importance for the faith system and/or their importance in the eyes of the deity, that faith system may, and in many cases does, contribute to individuals' feelings of self-worth. Where beliefs in an afterlife or reincarnation are part of the religion, what occurs in this life has an ultimate meaning that carries over into the next life or incarnation. What one believes, what one does, what one says, how one relates, are important but apart from the significance of actions, the individual is assured of divine attention and of meaning.

There is nothing particularly right or wrong about religious groups that provide meaning within their faith system, provided they do not insist that others conform to their beliefs and that others are granted the freedom to choose not to believe as they do. The socio-ethical guideline is freedom to choose insofar as that choice does not limit the rights and freedoms of others. It is when religious beliefs become "causes" that call for malevolent behavior toward others, insisting that meaning can be found in behavior that does violence to infidels or nonbelievers, that the ethical values inherent in a faith system break down. Freedom to protest publicly is acceptable, but when that freedom seeks to impose one set of beliefs on everyone, tries to inhibit freedom of choice, attempts to limit what others may read or see, or sets standards that thwart free expression, then any semblance of ethical standards or ethical behavior disappear. Destructive individuals may find meaning in their actions insofar as they believe they are fulfilling divine ordinances and acting as servants of their particular god, but that meaning becomes a twisted value statement in democratic settings.

One can be proud of elders who stand with picket signs expressing their religiously based approval or disapproval of actions by a government or by public officials. There can be no doubt that many are exhilarated and find meaning through identification with causes and in being associated with others who feel as they do. When the picket signs become weapons to injure others, whatever pride one may feel in elder action is replaced by disgust. The search for meaning can be, in part, an exciting participation in public action, when guided by reason, good judgment, understanding of human rights, and respect for the rights of those who differ. Without reason, causes can lead to local and international brutality, ranging from cruel harassment to war.

Certain groups of well-meaning believers can become nuisances when they confront busy travellers in airports and bus terminals. Others invade the privacy of homes by going from house to house peddling their beliefs and literature. Although most of these intruders are not elders, some are; these particular older persons seem to believe that gray hair and wrinkles should automatically guarantee respectful, listening audiences willing to yield their personal time to listen to presentations and perhaps arguments for a particular set of beliefs. Intrusion is intrusion whether practiced by young or old, and elders have no more right than others to trespass or encroach on another's time and privacy.

But what of those who do not subscribe to a religion or religious faith system? How do these elders find meaning? This leads us to the case of the cosmic orphan.

THE CASE OF THE COSMIC ORPHAN

There was a time when the cosmos had boundaries. Above was heaven—a solid firmament, the abode of the gods. Earth, which was conceived of as a flat disc, was the place of humans. Below was the grave, the place of the dead, or, according to some, the dwelling place of the demonic (Larue 1988). In those far-off days the gods were close, keeping watch over their created beings, evaluating behavior and rewarding or punishing as they saw fit. Temple ritual, literature, and the priesthood taught that the purpose of life was to fulfil the will of the gods, to serve them, and, of course, to support the priesthood as chosen servants of the gods. To the degree that these responsibilities were fulfilled, believers could be assured that their lives had meaning, and the obedient conformists were convinced that they were doing the right thing. If future rewards for fidelity to religious codes were promised, then the faithful could earn benefits in the afterlife, and ultimate meaning was to be found in eternal life in paradise. Of course meaning could be enhanced through satisfaction with what one did and by the praise one received as a true believer. The faith systems taught that life had purpose and meaning.

For most of us, these cosy images of the past are outmoded, despite the fact that some religious institutions continue to insist that they are relevant as divine revelations. Each of us is a creature of momentary existence in the millennia of time. As a species, we were not created to be servants of the gods; we evolved, as did all other living creatures. As individuals, we are the result of a single sexual encounter between our parents, which resulted in the chance union of one particular sperm with one particular ovum. We are creatures of happenstance, not of divine planning. God or the gods cannot be blamed or praised for who we are or what we are.

The cosmic view of our ancestors is not ours. We do not live in the enclosed space they envisioned. Instead, we live on a small chunk of cosmic matter that circles a small star in a universe of unimaginable dimensions.

Although life has not, as yet, been discovered elsewhere in the universe, there is a mathematical possibility that somewhere, on a planet far off in space, life forms have evolved that will, just as we are, be composed of the stuff of the universe. Should such life forms exist, they may have evolved along patterns similar to ours or they might be dramatically different.

As a consequence of our ever expanding knowledge, we humans have become cosmic orphans, lost in the vastness of time and space. Like single waves on a huge ocean, each one of us has a unique identity and significance in a moment of time before merging back in the whole. How can the cosmic orphan find meaning? The reactions vary.

Some find the cosmic reality overwhelming. They turn away from science and take refuge in teachings developed thousands of years ago before the development of science. They continue to deny evolution, despite the mounting evidence supporting the theory. They want to keep their heavens close so that they can claim their importance as creatures of a divine special creation.

Some accept the findings of science concerning the immensity of space and time and admit their infinitesimally small place in the cosmos. They may ponder the chance factors in their coming into being. At the same time, they cling to ancient faith systems. They box off their faith to keep it separate and apart from their scientific views. In other words, they live in two worlds—one scientific, the other religious—hoping that never the two shall meet. Many appear to live successful and happy lives. Meaning, for them, is still to be found in the faith system.

While some such bifurcated individuals maintain their divided thought patterns throughout life, others become troubled. Having accepted the implications of the scientific age and having moved away from ancient beliefs, they cannot find meaning in teachings that assure individuals of uniqueness and importance by insisting, for example, that even the hairs of the head are divinely numbered (Luke 12:7). Nor can such persons find a sense of personal meaning in boasts about how much their traditional faith system has contributed to the intellectual or moral history of humans. Such persons have abandoned the particularism of the past and embrace the universalism of today. Meaning has to be found elsewhere outside of the faith system. But where? Ultimately, for them as for all, the answer must be within the self (see below, "Meaning and the Inner Self"). However, some of these persons have developed positive statements—not as doctrines, but as affirmations of principles and values by which they live their lives. For example, in 1876, Felix Adler founded the Ethical Culture Societies, a religion that focuses on ethics rather than theology. Without denying or affirming belief in a god, Adler stated his understanding of human destiny as follows:

> We live in order to finish an, as yet, unfinished universe, unfinished so far as the human, that is, the highest part of it is concerned. We live in order to develop the superior qualities of man which are, as yet, for the most part latent. The test of genuine moral culture is to be found in the attention we pay to the oft-neglected details of conduct; in the extent to which we have formed the habit of asking, What is it right to do in those little things which yet are not so little? . . .
>
> We are to go out as teachers among the people, discarding the limitations of the past, and holding up the moral ideal, pure and simple, as the human ideal, as the ideal for all men, embracing all men, binding on all men—the ideal of a perfect society, of a society in which no men or class of men shall be mere hewers of wood and drawers of water for others; in which no man or woman, or class of men or class of women shall be used as tools for the lust of others, or for the ambitions of others, or for the greed of others; in which every human life, the life of every man and woman and child, shall be esteemed a sacred utterance of the Infinite. (Adler 1903, pp. 70–71)

His statement echoes ideals much like those of traditional religion but without references to a deity. Members find meaning as they participate in efforts to fulfill the founder's societal vision. Ethical culture groups formulate their own statements. The Ethical Culture Society of Los Angeles has stated its purpose as follows:

> Ethical Culture is a humanistic religious and educational movement inspired by the ideal that the supreme aim of human life is working to create a more humane society. Our faith is in the capacity and responsibility of human beings to act in their personal relationships and in the larger community to help create a better world.
>
> Our commitment is to the worth and dignity of the individual and to the treatment of each human being so as to bring out the best in him or her. Members join together in ethical ideals, to celebrate life's joys and support one another through life's crises, to work together to improve our world and the world of our children.*

Here the moral responsibilities of the individual and the organization are spelled out. Meaning is found in self-transformation and in efforts to change

---

*I found these statements on cards distributed by the Society.

society. Once again, many religious organizations would agree with the essence of these statements, adding only the concept of deity.

There are groups that eschew the term "religion" and describe themselves as "secular humanists." The "way" of humanism (Larue 1989) embraces a core of principles and values such as those that appear regularly on the back cover of *Free Inquiry*, a secular humanist magazine. It reads as follows:

> We are committed to the application of reason and science to the understanding of the universe and to the solving of human problems.
>
> We deplore efforts to denigrate human intelligence, to seek to explain the world in supernatural terms, and to look outside nature for salvation.
>
> We believe that scientific discovery and technology can contribute to the betterment of human life.
>
> We believe in an open and pluralistic society and that democracy is the best guarantee of protecting human rights from authoritarian elites and repressive majorities.
>
> We are committed to the principle of the separation of church and state.
>
> We cultivate the arts of negotiation and compromise as a means of resolving differences and achieving mutual understanding.
>
> We are concerned with securing justice and fairness in society and with eliminating discrimination and intolerance.
>
> We believe in supporting the disadvantaged and the handicapped so that they will be able to help themselves.
>
> We attempt to transcend divisive parochial loyalties based on race, religion, gender, nationality, creed, class, sexual orientation, or ethnicity, and strive to work together for the common good of humanity.
>
> We want to protect and enhance the earth, to preserve it for future generations, and to avoid inflicting needless suffering on other species.
>
> We believe in enjoying life here and now and in developing our creative talents to the fullest.
>
> We believe in the cultivation of moral excellence.
>
> We respect the right to privacy. Mature adults should be allowed to fulfill their aspirations, to express their sexual preferences, to exercise reproductive freedom, to have access to comprehensive and informed health care, and to die with dignity.
>
> We believe in the common moral decencies: altruism, integrity, honesty, truthfulness, responsibility. Humanist ethics is amenable to critical, rational guidance. There are normative standards that we discover together. Moral principles are tested by their consequences.
>
> We are deeply concerned with the moral education of our children. We want to nourish reason and compassion.

We are engaged by the arts no less than by the sciences.

We are citizens of the universe and are excited by the discoveries still to be made in the cosmos.

We are skeptical of untested claims to knowledge, and we are open to novel ideas and seek new departures in our thinking.

We affirm humanism as a realistic alternative to theologies of despair and ideologies of violence and as a source of rich personal significance and genuine satisfaction in the service of others.

We believe in optimism rather than pessimism, hope rather than despair, learning in the place of dogma, truth instead of ignorance, joy rather than guilt or sin, tolerance in the place of fear, love instead of hatred, compassion over selfishness, beauty instead of ugliness, and reason rather than blind faith or irrationality.

We believe in the fullest realization of the best and noblest that we are capable of as human beings.

This overlong *credo* seeks to embrace all dimensions of life and implies that secularists find meaning insofar as they are able to live up to or conform to the enunciated principles. Once again, many of the basic concepts are not unlike those accepted by major religions and, once again, the difference lies in the absence of a belief in a deity. However, like the religious believer, the humanist must also look beyond doing and thinking to the person within to discover the self and the meaning of the self.

MEMORY

Interestingly enough, many elders never attempt to assess the meaning or significance of their own lives. In a casual way, they may relate meaning to work done or to family ties, but not to the self. No self-probing has been undertaken to enable them to discover the inner self, that core of the person which relates experience to feelings of self-esteem and self-confidence or, on the contrary, to feelings of defeat or deprivation, frustration or despair.

Erik Erikson has described the tensions within the psyche in old age as being between integrity and despair. The term "integrity"

seems to describe the aging individual's struggles to integrate the strength and purpose necessary to maintain wholeness despite disintegrating physical capacities. It also suggests the need to gather the experiences of a long and eventful life into a meaningful pattern. (Erikson, Erikson, and Kivnick 1986, p. 288)

Despair is also an ingredient in the psyche's "struggle for balance":

> To have experienced the world and our human inadequacy to deal with
> one another and our mutual problems in living and growing is consistently
> to know defeat. To balance the pull of despair, which may well increase
> with waning strength, we need to muster all the ingredients of the wisdom
> we have been garnering throughout the life stages. (Erikson, Erickson,
> and Kivnick 1986, p. 288)

The reconciliation of these tensions lies in the integrating potential and
strength of wisdom. Wisdom confirms the validity of relationships and
experiences and continues to draw the person into involvement with life
and living. What is the basis of this wisdom and how is this achieved?

Wisdom, according to Erikson, includes everything from "ripened 'wits'
to accumulated knowledge and matured judgment. It is the essence of
knowledge freed of temporal relativity" (Erikson 1964, p. 133). He continues:
"*Wisdom, then, is detached concern with life itself, in the face of death
itself.*"* It is this matured, detached wisdom that enables the elder to make
contributions to the future.

The elements of that mature wisdom include, at the very least: hope,
will, and fidelity. Hope, as opposed to hopelessness, anticipates the future
and keeps open the doors of choice. It is a positive, life-enhancing stance
as opposed to hopelessness in which no potentials for choice can be imagined.
Will embraces the feeling and intention of self-determination and control,
which is also a positive mental posture. Fidelity involves being true to
what one has been, still is and will continue to be. The integration of
the self is the outcome of such inner commitments to life as opposed
to despair.

Although Erikson's postulates sound as if one needs a course in
developmental psychology and, perhaps, also philosophy before they can
be grasped, wisdom in old age has no such prerequisites. The wise elder
is the one who has lived through the dramatic transitions in lifestyle and
fortune described earlier in this book and who can, to some degree, make
sense of what has happened and what is happening. Such a person maintains
poise within the maelstrom of life's swirling changes to find direction and
perhaps meaning in existence. Time is a prerequisite for such thinking
and perhaps also freedom from extreme pain and poverty. What is most
important, is that insofar as society recognizes the importance of the elder's

---

*Emphasis is in the original.

self-integration, provision should be made to enable elders to reach this final stage of self-actualization. It is when health breaks down and pain becomes constant, or when poverty reduces living to bare existence, that despair or depression and feelings of meaninglessness dominate. At that stage, many elders are prepared to abandon courage (see chapter 18) to give up on life and choose death (see chapter 19).

REMEMBERING FOR THE FUTURE

Can memory contribute to meaning? Emphasis has been placed on the importance memories hold for elders. It has been suggested that through recall some elders are able to assess the meaning of their lives. But there is another dimension to elder memory; it is remembering for the future.

Modern youth can discover details of the past through history books, through novels, through television documentaries and through visits to museums and period houses. A different dimension is to be found in elder memory and it relates to the future—a future that may have significance for members of a single family or for the whole human family. What lessons have been learned? What insights have been gained? How does the past relate to the present and to what lies ahead?

One young female student, recovering from a painful divorce, was given an assignment to talk with her mother about the mother's wedding. She was not too enthusiastic about the idea because neither her marriage nor her divorce had been acceptable in her rather conservative family. The first interview took place when her mother was in the kitchen, pressing lace doilies. The student took notes and tape recorded the conversation. As they talked, the father, who had been listening from the living room, entered the kitchen and said, "That's not the way I remembered it." The student had been estranged from her father but in the kitchen setting, conversation flowed.

Subsequently, she was given parental diaries and bundles of love letters to read. Her research led her to her maternal grandmother and once again, in addition to talking, she read love letters and documents that augmented memories. She uncovered in these two female progenitors what she called a "feistiness and independence of spirit" that was akin to what she felt in herself. In what they had written, she found kinship of feelings and responses to parallel life situations. She discovered a familial heritage that contributed to her growing sense of self-identity and that encouraged confidence in herself and her ability to survive, just as her mother and grandmother had survived family tensions, war, poverty, losses, illnesses, and deaths. None of this could she have derived from books that described the past in general, nor from popular "how to" books that advised how one should face divorce, separation, or life in general. Only through the shared words, memories, and records of her family heritage was this student given insight into a personal legacy that was uniquely hers. This provided guidance and perhaps a vision pertaining to who she might become.

This is not to suggest that the past has no broader meaning for the present or for the future. The development of centers of research and memories concerning the Holocaust have demonstrated the importance of remembering that horrendous human experiment in extermination. Those involved in the preservation of memories of that event find meaning in the knowledge that the recounting of what they saw, heard, felt, and recalled becomes part of human history. How they coped and how they survived become lessons in human courage, compassion, and cooperation. Their survival is not meaningless, nor are the deaths of those who did not survive without significance. What is most important is that the records serve as a warning for the future. They keep us aware of the potential for evil in humans and in human society. They probe responses to that evil as we attempt to understand how Germany—a great, civilized nation that had produced outstanding philosophers, writers, artists, poets, psychologists, and humanitarians—could, almost overnight, degenerate into a cruel, destructive, and, some would say, demonic state. The examination of the responses of those who survived provide us with clues to survival patterns that are both demeaning and ennobling. Most of all, these memories serve as a warning to present and future generations that lurking beneath the thin veneer of civilization are the shadowy but destructive forces of bigotry, racism, and prejudice of one kind or another, including agism. We are safe so long as we remember and commit ourselves to the preservation of a life of dignity and safety for all. What more ennobling and exciting task could be set before any elder or group of elders? Who they were and who they are truly matters.

Similar projects are being undertaken with regard to the millions slaughtered under the regime of Joseph Stalin in Russia, and with the Afro-American, Latino, Japanese, and other similar groups' experiences in America. The theme is "Remember! Do not forget!" Indeed, such memories provide assurance that no life was shed in vain, no suffering was meaningless, since out of the ashes of the past the phoenix of the future must rise.

On a less dramatic scale, familial memories are being recorded. Elders are asked "What would you like to say to your great, great grandchildren who will never know you in person and whom you will never see? Will you tell them what it was like to grow up in your time, how you found your first job, what you wore at your wedding, your reactions at the birth of a child, and so on and on?" War memories, depression-period recollections, stories of losses and victories in one's life help to define who the person is; such definitions give meaning to the self. Moreover, they give a historical identity to the family.

Consider the example of an elder who has retired from his life work before his wife retired from hers. He is restless, fretful, and fusses at busy work that simply adds to his feelings of meaninglessness. He came alive when we talked of his rich background of experiences in life, of his insights and perceptions, of how what he did contributed to the development of modern culture. But then the light dimmed and he lapsed into his feelings of irritation at what he had become. The light went on again when he was persuaded that he had something to leave as a heritage. Now, through recording his memoirs, his great, great grandchildren, whom he will never see, will have access to his innermost thoughts, his voice, and his character. He will no longer be just a name on the family tree. His retired time is no longer useless. Indeed, he now sits at a word processor and puts his thoughts on a diskette before he reads them into a recorder. He continues to discover things in himself and about himself that he wants to share. He is, in fact, in a process of self-discovery, of integrating the self. He tended to be a bit preachy when he began, but he soon moved beyond that phase and has become an autobiographer who enjoys where he has been in life and what he is sharing. What this man did can set an example for any elder.

WHEN THE LIGHT GROWS DIM

What happens to those for whom the sense of meaning or purpose has gone out of life? What do elders do when suddenly they are no longer employed or employable, when time rests heavily upon them and they have no significant responsibilities other than those associated with mere survival? How do they cope?

It is possible to approach these questions with a set of "oughts." These individuals *ought* to have prepared for retirement years with meaningful events to fill the time. They all *ought* to engage in autobiographical writing. There are volunteer activities with which retired elders *ought* to become involved. Such quick solutions to boredom may have validity, but they ignore the feeling many elders have that their rich repositories of skills, wisdom, and ability are no longer important to a society that places its elderly on the discard heap. Older adults have become part of the "no deposit, no return" mentality that fills our waste piles with materials that in earlier times would have been recycled and put to significant use. Unlike bottles, cans, and paper, there is precious little recycling of human potential. The consequences of such rejection include expanded social and financial burdens associated with the health problems of elders, many of which are directly related to feelings of social uselessness and helplessness.

My grandfather was retired at the age of seventy. He owned his home. His wife had died thirty-five years earlier but his eldest daughter, who lived with him, cared for the home and provided companionship. For the past quarter of a century his life had followed a regular routine. He rose each morning at 6:00, washed, shaved, ate breakfast, and walked to St. Mary's Cathedral where he attended Mass at 7:00. His workday began at 8:30 at the city Street Car "barns" where he repaired the windows in trolley cars, some of which had been broken by wayward youngsters like myself. He was an expert craftsman and had devised techniques that replaced the windows with precisely cut panes and without damage to the sashes. He was proud of his work, happy with what he was doing, at ease with his fellow workers, and content with his lifestyle.

Each evening he walked home, arriving about 6:00, washed up, changed clothes, and ate his dinner. He read the evening paper with his favorite cat purring contentedly on his lap. On Saturdays he cared for the lawns, his garden, and his greenhouse. On Sunday, dressed in his best clothes, he walked with his daughter to the church, attended Mass, came home, read the Sunday paper, and spent the day quietly in conversation with friends. Monday was always a welcome day, it marked the beginning of his work week.

Then suddenly he was retired. There was nothing wrong with his work, but he had reached the age of seventy, and even this was an extension of the usual retirement age. On the first day of his retirement, he rose at 6:00 A.M., washed, ate breakfast, attended 7:00 A.M. Mass, and then went to the Car Barns. There was a new employee, a young man, in the workroom he had designed. This newcomer abandoned my grandfather's tested methods and was less concerned about protection of window sashes. My grandfather shared his wisdom and puttered about the work areas talking and interfering with the established work patterns of others. After one week of such visits, my aunt received phone calls asking that "the old man" be kept away. This was not easy. Ultimately he accepted the necessary change, and after morning mass he began to wander the streets, looking in windows, just passing the time. He was bored. He was lost, and he felt useless. Disorientation set in. He become lost on the streets of his city; time and again the police brought him home, until they, too, requested that something be done to keep him closer to home. His disorientation increased. Soon his wandering changed as he imagined that he was back in his boyhood home and sought to find places he once knew in a far off province. He was labelled senile. Within three-and-a-half years he was dead. Grandfather simply gave up on life. This once healthy, vigorous working man was no longer needed by the society he had helped develop. He was now useless, discarded. In his day there were no senior centers. His church had not developed programs for the elderly. He became a lost soul who did not cope well—so he died.

There are those who have suggested that "disengagement" is a normal, natural, inevitable part of the aging process (Cumming and Henry 1961). In disengagement one willingly lets go of social involvement and, of course, for those elders who are vegetating in mental institutions disengagement might seem to be a reasonable option. But for the vast majority, like my grandfather, there is a decided preference for participation in significant social roles. Without such involvement, life becomes a meaningless existence that they feel helpless to change. Growing old poses an existential problem, an ethical issue, that society dare not ignore.

MEANING THROUGH OFFSPRING

The cartoonist Irving Lazarus, creator of "Momma," often portrays elders seeking, finding, or attempting to find meaning in the roles of their offspring. Momma's friends all seem to have successful sons and daughters who follow profitable professions or who have married into socially acceptable and rich families. These elders apparently see themselves as beyond finding meaning in their own lives so they seek meaning in the roles and positions of their children.

Momma often exalts her own status by criticism of her daughter-in-law, demeaning the younger woman's cooking and house-cleaning. She tries to persuade her one successful, married son to return to her home, to an environment where (according to her) the food is better and the house is cleaner. She exalts her role by derogating her youngest son who is in rebellion against the work ethic. He is depicted as a rather useless young man, devoid of ambition and dependent upon Momma's handouts and free room and board. Any prospective date or mate he presents to Momma is dismissed as some kind of "bimbo" or as lacking in brain-power. Similar evaluations are made of the daughter's boyfriends. Momma exalts herself at the expense of others. She copes with meaninglessness by seeking to control and by demeaning others.

Even the older men who approach Momma with any kind of romantic intentions are depicted as semi-senile, lacking in energy, feeble, or otherwise unacceptable. Lazarus's depiction of elders implies that these rather silly old people find much of their meaning and purpose in putting down others—a most unfortunate caricature, and one which is not, fortunately, the dominant reality.

On the other hand, Lazarus is correct when he implies that some elders do find meaning in the accomplishments of their children. The research by the Eriksons and Kivnick (1986, pp. 75ff) disclosed parents who took personal pride in their children's parenting and housekeeping skills as well as in their academic and professional attainments. Indeed familial pride can extend to incorporate the classroom successes of grandchildren. Some years ago, a friend spent a sabbatic leave at Harvard University, where he was engaged in research. When he returned he commented that faculty prestige and prowess were not based on degrees or publications, since every professor seemed to have an abundance of those symbols of success. What appeared to matter most were the grades one's children received in school. If his observation was correct, one can only imagine the impossible burden placed on the children who became responsible for parental social status!

MEANING AND SERVICE

Elders were taught to serve; they were not of the "me generation." As children, they were part of a family in which household tasks were divided and they were expected to "pull their weight." As they matured into their teens, many held part-time jobs: delivering newspapers, cutting lawns, shovelling snow, selling magazines door-to-door, and so on. Part of what they earned went into family coffers. They were taught familial responsibility. When they married and had families, they engaged in various parental roles as den mothers, members of Parent Teachers Associations, voters' leagues, church programs, and the like.

Now, as elders, they have not stopped. Many belong to service organizations or are volunteers for local programs ranging from ecological

was a bit dopey (she was unconscious) from her medicine. When the son left work in the evening and came to visit, his mother was dead. Jake died one week after the funeral.

For Eva, death was preferable to living as a handicapped person. Her past made it too difficult for her to cope with her present and with the increasing disability and dependency she saw ahead. She exercised choice and committed suicide. Jake's death was no surprise. I had warned the son that his father was frail and was dependent on Eva's company. After his father's funeral, the son wondered if his father had not clung to life so that Eva would continue to have the financial benefits that came from Jake's retirement policy. When she died, his reason for living was gone.

Eva's choice of suicide was not one that others might make. There are many elders who continue to find meaning in life despite handicaps far more severe and burdensome than Eva's. But the choice was hers, and in the light of what was known of her damaged childhood, one can understand her decision, whether or not one approves of it.

Betty, on the other hand, adapts to limitations. She doesn't like the crippling arthritis and her dependency on drugs to control pain, but she has found much to live for. Her granddaughter is an important person in Betty's life and the opportunity to encourage the twelve-year-old to explore varying dimensions of living is Betty's delight. In addition to caring for her pet dog, Betty has a neighbor, Bertha, who is also old and crippled. They have developed a daily exchange of newspapers that involves the exercise of a slow, shuffling walk across the street separating their two houses. Nieces and nephews love Betty's relaxed attitude toward life and visit when they come to town. Her youngest brother (also retired) who lives 200 miles away visits every other week. Her oldest brother, who lives across the continent, phones several times per month. When her pain becomes severe and she cannot sleep, Betty rises in the darkness of the early morning and writes letters to relatives far and near. Hers is a limited life—severely limited—but she entertains no thoughts of suicide. Her childhood and her marriage were not easy but it never scarred her with inner unhealed wounds like those of Eva.

If anything comes through from these two brief case histories, it is that we are all different and therefore our choices in adapting to the limitations imposed by aging and ailing bodies will differ. Each choice must be accepted without condemnation, for our ethic must embrace the wisdom embodied in an old Indian saying that we should never judge the behavior of another until we have walked a mile in his or her moccasins. For Eva, meaning was gone; for Betty, meaning is alive and well.

LOVE ADDS MEANING

Perhaps for most of us, the most significant contributor to meaning is the capacity to love and be loved. To be loved by another is to be accepted, appreciated, deemed important, and given meaning. To love and to be able to give significance to another (or others) through love gives importance and identity to the life of both the lover and the beloved. To be without love is to be lonely and isolated from others and compelled to find meaning elsewhere.

Some elders are not easy to love. They are insensitive, judgmental, harsh, bitter, angry, or hostile. They make cruel remarks and belittle others as they seek to enhance their own poor self-evaluation. They never praise without adding words of criticism ("You look nice, *but* . . ."). They demand recognition that others may feel they have not earned and do not deserve. When the recognition is given, it is not appreciated. They become disruptive factors in a community or nursing home and can be thoroughly disliked by most everyone. For such persons, love is negated as a significant source of meaning because such elders do not know how to love.

Fortunately, those who are hard to be with are in the minority. Most elders are ready and willing to give love, and they appreciate love in return. The bonds that unite a couple who have lived and loved together for decades cannot be underestimated, and it is not surprising to find that when one mate dies, the other, most often the male (as in the case of Jake) dies soon after.

WHEN THE LIGHT GOES OUT

It was noted above that the brain is the organ of meaning. When the brain ceases to function rationally, due to some disease such as Alzheimer's, or due to an accident or illness that places the individual in a vegetative state, then for that person, all sense of meaning is greatly diminished or is completely gone. Through the love and affectionate responses of caregivers, the person with diminished reasoning capacities may be conscious of being cared for and may grasp the importance of being loved, but a rational sense of meaning other than, perhaps a fuzzy awareness of "I matter because I am loved" is not present. Of course, the important relationship between love and meaning cannot be dismissed, no matter how faintly recognized.

MEANING AND THE INNER SELF

In most of the ways discussed above by which elders achieve meaning, the point of reference was external to the self. That is to say, they find meaning in what they do and in the acceptance of worth conveyed in the eyes of others. People find meaning in family and in how the family accepts and approves of them. Meaning can also be found through religion or altruistic service. In each instance, elders look outside of the self for acceptance, for approval, for recognition.

Some years ago a wise old church member embarrassed his minister with lavish praise for work done. His explanation was simple, "I don't believe in sending flowers to a funeral. I prefer to present them when a person is alive!" For most of us, the plaudits, the accolades, the words of praise related to what we have done or what we have signified are spoken at our funerals or memorial services, which we cannot hear or appreciate. Without thoughtful individuals like the wise old church member to help us understand the meaning of our lives, where do we turn for guidance?

The most important provider of meaning must be the self—the independent, not the dependent, self. To evaluate who and what one is purely on the basis of external recognition denies the validity of self-evaluation. Meaning-filled persons live satisfying lives not because some outside source tells them that their lives have meaning (as pleasant and fulfilling as that may be), but because of inner certitude. The feelings must come from inside as one looks back and evaluates where one has been, what one has experienced, who one has affected.

Unfortunately, self-appreciation is difficult for many adults. We have been taught that it is an evil, a vice, and socially impolite or improper to feel good about oneself. "Ego trips," as they are sometimes called, are deemed insufferable. We are encouraged to think not about ourselves but about "others." Altruism is preferable to healthy self-concern. "Self-pride" or "vanity," which is used to symbolize the idolizing of the self, can be interpreted as pathological narcissism and labelled "asocial" (Fromm 1964, ch. 4).

But there is another point of view. Both self-esteem and pride can be evaluated positively. According to Nathaniel Brandon,

Self-esteem . . . pertains to an inner conviction of our fundamental efficacy and worth. Pride pertains to the more explicitly conscious pleasure we take in ourselves on the basis of and in response to specific achievements or actions. Positive self-esteem is "I can." Pride is "I have," and the deepest pride we can experience is that which results from the achievement of self-esteem, for self-esteem is a value that has to be earned—and has to be maintained.

Pride is a positive emotional experience, just as self-esteem is. It is not a vice to overcome but a virtue to be attained—a form of honoring the self. (1983, p. 15)

From infancy many of us are encouraged to rely upon others for acceptance. Inner certitude begins to develop early and is affected by environment; it can be hindered and retarded by associations. When little children are taught to depend on adult approval for their sense of meaning, when they are scolded, condemned, put down, spanked, and slapped for self-expression or for revealing their feelings, they begin to learn that feelings are secondary, not to be trusted, and, perhaps, invalid. When a child speaks up, interrupts, or cries out against something that is happening only to be reproved, ignored, or punished for that personal reaction, the youngster is being told that there is something amiss with his or her feelings and their expression. Children soon learn not to trust their own appraisals and to look to others for evaluation of the self and for validation of ideas.

A quick look inside a classroom will reveal how insecure persons become with their own ability to evaluate. When university students are presented with a scholarly essay and asked to react to and evaluate what the author says, the tendency is to report on *what* the writer has stated, rather than employ a critical or analytical approach. These young people are insecure about the validity of their own thinking and responses.

Feelings of self-doubt and personal inadequacy can remain locked in place providing the adult with a child's view of the self and the universe. W. Hugh Missildine writes of *Your Inner Child of the Past* (1963):

The child you once were continues to survive inside your adult shell. "Thrive" would perhaps be a better word than "survive," for often this "inner child of the past" is a sprawling, bawling, brawling character—racing pell-mell into activities he likes, upsetting and wrecking others' lives—or perhaps the child is the fearful, timid, shrinking part of your personality.

Whether we like it or not, we are simultaneously the child we once were, who lives in the emotional atmosphere of the past and often interferes in the present, and an adult who tries to forget the past and live wholly in the present. The child you once were can balk or frustrate your adult satisfactions, embarrass and harass you, make you sick—or enrich your life. (p. 14)

He observes, "Much distress, fatigue, loneliness, and inner emptiness could be eliminated if people had a deeper understanding of how to live fruitfully with their 'inner child of the past' " (p. 16).

Leah was born in Greece. She has a distressing memory of childhood that has haunted her throughout her sixty-nine years of life. She was the last of seven children and her mother informed her over and over again, "You are a cursed child" because the mother was unable to bear children after Leah's birth. One might dismiss the mother's statement as an angry response from a woman who found her identity in bearing many children. To Leah it became the inner child who contributed to an insecurity that she masked as a successful mother and wife able to function admirably in society. But the inner child was there and it spoke to the mature woman with the voice of parental authority: "You are cursed!"

Freeing Leah from the powerful control of the inner child was both painful and exhilarating. She had to be led to the point where, in her mind, she could visualize that child she once was—alone, isolated, forlorn, devastated by the mother's indictment, and made frightened and insecure. What a sad and tear-filled moment of recognition! She had to take that child into her arms (mentally), embrace it, claim it, reassure it that it was not cursed, and love it for itself. Then, in her mind, taking the hand of the child, she walked away from the past—down the road to where it bent. At that place, she bade farewell to her mother (long dead) and to the language and the curse that had haunted her, turned the corner to find herself with her accepted child-self on a new road, free from the past that she could no longer visualize, because it was left on the old roadway. Sounds simple? Not really! The process is neither easy nor rapid. It requires work with a therapist. It churns up feelings of pain and produces tears as one confronts the injured child. But it brings excitement and exhilaration as the adult is freed of the battered child's control. It permits the inner child to become the adult. The process begins with the recognition of the inner child affecting the adult.

There are many adults who as children experienced supportive reactions to their expressions of feeling and whose opinions were treated with respect.

These fortunate ones tend to find meaning within themselves. They are sure of who they are and what they are. They matter because they have always mattered. Their life has meaning because it has always had meaning.

Most of the time, we are too much in a hurry, too busy, to probe the background of elders to find what does and does not provide meaning in their lives. The film *It's a Wonderful Life,* which is usually shown on television during the winter solstice, gives an individual (George Bailey, played by Jimmy Stewart) an opportunity to see what life would have been like if he had never existed, thereby providing insight into the ways his individual life affected others. The solstice is an appropriate time for presenting the film, for although many elders find the family gatherings and gift-giving exciting and exhilarating, others are depressed. The shortened hours of daylight and the longer hours of darkness shed an aura of gloom. Some experience extreme loneliness and feelings of isolation at this time of the year. Gifts become trivia and family gatherings less than joyous. It becomes important for the media to present entertainment that suggests ways in which elders (and others) can look back over their lives and into themselves to recognize the fact that in their own way they have made a difference.

There is nothing particularly unethical in self-esteem and self-pride despite what some religions, some families, and some ethicists teach. Both can be healthy enablers to the search for personal meaning. What is unethical is a religion or a society that insists that one must always place the importance and significance of others before the self.

REFERENCES

Adler, Felix. 1903. *Life and Destiny.* New York: McClure, Phillips & Co.

Bettelheim, Bruno. 1976. *The Uses of Enchantment.* New York: Alfred A. Knopf.

Branden, Nathaniel. 1970. *The Psychology of Self-Esteem.* New York: Bantam Books.

———. 1983. *Honoring the Self.* Los Angeles: Jeremy P. Tarcher, Inc.

Cumming, Elaine, and William E. Henry. 1961. *Growing Old: The Process of Disengagement.* New York: Basic Books.

Erikson, Erik H. 1964. *Insight and Responsibility.* New York: W. W. Norton and Co.

Erikson, Erik H., Joan M. Erikson, and Helen Q. Kivnick. 1986. *Vital Involvement in Old Age.* New York: W. W. Norton and Co.

Finkelstein, Louis. 1949, 1955. "The Jewish Religion: Its Beliefs and Practices," in Louis Finkelstein, ed., *The Jews: Their History, Culture, and Religion,* Vol. II, New York: Harper and Row, pp. 1327–43.

Fromm, Erich. 1964. *The Heart of Man: Its Genius for Good and Evil.* New York: Harper and Row.

Larue, Gerald A. 1988. *Ancient Myth and Modern Life.* Long Beach, Calif.: Centerline Press.

———. 1989. *The Way of Ethical Humanism.* Long Beach, Calif.: Centerline Press.

———. 1989. *The Way of Positive Humanism.* Long Beach, Calif.: Centerline Press.

Lasch, Christopher. 1979. *The Culture of Narcissism.* New York: W. W. Norton, and Warner Books, Inc.

Missildine, W. Hugh. 1963. *Your Inner Child of the Past.* New York: Simon and Schuster.

Troll, L. E., S. J. Miller, and R. C. Atchley. 1979. *Families in Later Life.* Belmont, Calif.: Wadsworth.

11

Geroethics and Longevity

"In a sense, longevity is the measure of the individual's ability to cope with an ever changing environment."

—Johnson, *Relations Between Normal Aging and Disease*, p. viii

Once upon a time, in the good old days, people lived long, long lives. Or did they?

The human dream of long life has a long history of its own and is expressed in our earliest literature. The Sumerians wrote about those wonderful old times when kings ruled for eons—En-men-lu-Anna for 43,200 years, Alalgar for 36,000 years, Alulium for 28,800 years, and so on. As the ancient king list approached the time when the document was written, reality set in and the length of sovereignty was dramatically reduced; Mes-kiag-Nanna reigned twenty-five years and Balulu thirty-six years (Larue 1985).

A similar pattern appears in the biblical record of pre-flood heroes. Methuselah lived for 969 years, Lamech 777 years, and his son Noah 950 years, during which, at age 500, he fathered three sons and, when he was 600 years old, he built an ark (Gen. 5–9)! Of course, the Sumerian and biblical records are fiction designed to bridge gaps in history concerning which ancient writers had no knowledge. No one was ever so long-lived, but the dream was always there.

Even the story of the patriarch Abraham and his wife Sarah is an obvious exaggeration. At the age of eighty-six, Abraham sired his first child by Hagar, Sarah's Egyptian maid (Gen. 16:15). When he was 100 and Sarah was 90, they produced a child, Isaac (Gen. 17:1–18:15; 21:1–

132

5). After Sarah died, Abraham, at age 135, married Keturah (who was probably in her teens) and produced more offspring (Gen. 25:1-4). He is supposed to have died at age 175 (Gen 25:7). One can see that Abraham could readily become a hero figure for male elders!

Sarah, too, has distinct possibilities as a heroine for the female elder group. When she was sixty-five, she was so strikingly beautiful that she became a member of Pharaoh's harem (Gen. 12:15). Centuries later, Jewish monastics living on the shores of the Dead Sea described her beauty in these terms: "Her face is beautiful and how fine are her tresses! How lovely are her eyes! How delicate is her nose and the entire sheen of her face! How well-formed are her breasts and how fair her complexion! How pleasing are her arms and how perfect her hands! How desirable are her hands to look at and how long and slender her fingers! How dainty are her feet and how shapely are her thighs! None of the virgins or brides that enter the marriage chamber is more beautiful than she! She is fairer than all other women; her beauty is greater than theirs" (see Gaster 1976, p. 365; Vermes 1973, p. 218). Now obviously, these desert-dwelling monastics, most of whom appear to have been celibate, let their fantasies and imaginations run free, as they added to the idealization of the sixty-five-year-old Sarah. Their comments support the conviction of many modern elders that beauty need not fade with age.

The desire for long life and the fiction of patriarchal longevity did not negate reality thinking; the brevity of human existence was admitted. The ancient legend concerning the search for immortality by King Gilgamesh of Uruk, discussed earlier, ended in frustration for he, despite his human-divine status, was doomed to die like every other mortal (Larue 1988, pp. 85-90). Even when he acquired the miraculous rejuvenation plant that would "make the old man young," its benefits were denied him when the plant was devoured by a snake. Thus, the serpent, too, was enabled to shed its aging skin and renew itself, while (alas) humans must simply wrinkle with age. The biblical myth of the garden of Eden has a similar motive—the first humans failed to eat of the tree of immortality before they were ejected, therefore human life is limited. A Psalmist believed that seventy years of age constituted longevity and that eighty years of age was to be taken as symbolic of vigor:

> Our life span is 70 years,
> 80 at most, if we are strong,
> and they pass quickly in troublesome work,
> ere we drift away. (Ps. 90:10)

Although tradition taught that the elders of the past lived dramatically long lives, there were those who confronted the facts and recorded what they knew.

During the Middle Ages, alchemists were fascinated with the potential of the salamander to regenerate a severed tail. If only they could discover the secret of that process, perhaps they could discover a way to regenerate failing humans and extend life. Of course they failed.

But the search for longevity has continued. Modern studies have produced new fiction concerning long-lived groups. At one time the villagers of Vilacambamba in the Ecuadorian Andes, the Hunzas of Kashmir, and the Abkhazians in the former Soviet Union were hailed as humans who not only became centenarians without loss of vigor, but some were supposed to have reached ages as high as 150 years. Recent investigations have cast doubt on these claims. There is no question that significant numbers of old people live in these communities but they have not reached the ages once claimed for them. Because there is almost no reliance on high technologies and mechanized patterns of travel, these elders walk more and engage in activities that contribute to their physical fitness. Their diet, made up of unrefined products with an abundance of vegetables and grains, also appears to contribute to health and longevity. The elders tend to be sexually active and their social environment provides psychological support. No doubt genetic heritage is also involved. The claims to excessively long lives no longer stands, but the evidence of vigorous elders does (Pelletier 1982, pp. 282–318).

What can be documented is that between 1969 and 1979 the number of centenarians in the United States rose from 3,000 to more than 10,000 (Pepper 1979) and estimates indicate that by the year 2000, the number of persons over 100 years old will have increased to more than 100,000.

PERHAPS WE CAN SLOW THE AGING PROCESS

Modern researchers continue to seek ways to delay aging and extend life. For example, one study that involved the reduction of body temperature in lower life forms for periods of time (hypothermia) as well as controlling the diet, suggested that temperature and diet might be factors in increasing the life span. Others have looked to miracle drugs and biochemical responses to new pharmaceuticals that offer some promise of altering the aging process. Daniel Rudman of the Medical College of Wisconsin and the Veterans Affairs Medical Center in Milwaukee reported that injections of human growth hormone (HGH) made the bodies of twenty-three elderly men more youthful and actually reversed some aspects of the aging process. The lean body tissue of the men increased 9 percent and their fat tissue decreased 14 percent, reversing the normal pattern of loss of lean body tissue due to aging. The possible long-term effects of this expensive process ($14,000 per year) are unknown, but it is known that HGH can stimulate abnormal bone growth (Vreeland 1990). Neuroscientists have looked to the brain for answers to longevity. Most recently experts in cell biology are raising hopes for the possible "re-education" of body cells responsible for aging, in the hope of extending life. Genetic research may provide means to thwart disease and disabilities associated with aging; it would program genes, which, when combined with sensible diet and exercise, could greatly expand the human life span.

CAN WE CHANGE THE APPEARANCE OF AGING?

Some present-day elders would be pleased if they could change or reverse the appearance of aging—that is, they would like to look younger than they really are (the Sarah syndrome?). The desire is not new. Like modern elders, ancient people sought to deter or to eliminate the signs of aging. For example, the Egyptians prepared their own mixtures to prevent gray hair. One recipe called for the womb of a cat warmed in oil and mixed with the egg of a gabgu bird. Another included a roasted hoof of an ass, a dog's vulva, a black tapeworm, plus a worm found in dung, mixed with oil and gum and rubbed on the scalp (Bryan 1974, p. 155). Wrinkles were treated for six days with a combination of incense cake, wax, fresh olive oil, Cyperus, and fresh milk (Bryan, p. 158). It is likely that these ancient forms of hair coloring and retin-A were no more effective than their modern counterparts in effacing the signs of aging. Certainly their ingredients would not come under present day pharmaceutical regulations!

Although there are some elders who scorn the efforts, there is nothing unethical in the efforts to erase or slow the signs of aging. Why not do all that one can to look one's best? What is unethical is the exploitation of the fears of aging by those who advertise and sell products that may be harmless but which fail to live up to the publicized promises and do nothing to erase wrinkles or the signs of aging.

Some nonmedicinal efforts are just a little amusing. One woman decided that smiling kept the face muscles from sagging. She wore a perpetual smile, even enduring the most trying situations. Unfortunately, her face sagged and jowls appeared. In truth, she gave the image of a happy person and perhaps brightened the scene a bit, but what lay behind the smile was a futile effort to defeat the forces of gravity and age.

Another woman tried an almost diametrically opposed facial exercise. She decided to keep her face calm. The last time I saw her, she had an almost mask-like appearance, fortified now by heavy make-up that seemed to me to be supporting her face! She seemed to be afraid to smile (lest the make-up crack?).

Of course there are operations that change appearances. Face-lifts are not uncommon and some men and women have had as many as three or four, each seeking to pull and stretch the sagging skin to keep the face free of wrinkles and jowls. Tummy-tucks reduce waistlines just as implants and other breast surgeries reshape the bustline. Unfortunately and unhappily, there are a few unethical and improperly trained surgeons who perform such operations and who botch the job. Patients, including elders, are scarred for the rest of their lives, much to the dismay of insurance companies and to the satisfaction of lawyers.

LONGEVITY AND MAY-DECEMBER MARRIAGES

Marriages between elders and younger men or women are not uncommon and are sometimes interpreted as efforts on the part of the elder to recapture youth. Such unions are commonly labelled "May-December" marriages by a skeptical public.

Looking at the May-December marriages of well-known movie personalities such as Charlie Chaplin or Fred Astaire, and government officials like Strom Thurmond, there is clear evidence that many of these unions seem to work. There is no real evidence that the elder is seeking to become younger and obviously the elder does not become more youthful, nor does the younger partner age more rapidly. Inasmuch as I am personally in a May-December marriage, I know that what lies behind my own most wonderful relationship is not any effort on my part to deny my aging, but simply a love that has grown in quality, depth, and intensity year by year and even day by day. Therefore, if my own experience provides any clue to other marriages that ignore age differences, there is, perhaps, a greater awareness of age and less denial of age and only the wish that there could be more time ahead for the elder partner. And when two people love one another and marry for love, there are no ethical issues involved.

LIVING LONGER DOES NOT GUARANTEE LIVING BETTER

Suppose that scientists do find ways to enable humans to gain an extra twenty or thirty or fifty years to reach age 120 or even 130. Is the expanded time desirable if the quality of life is not simultaneously enhanced?

The Greeks realized that immortality or extended longevity in and of itself is not enough. The Homeric *Hymn to Aphrodite* (eighth century B.C.E.) tells of the love between the dawn goddess Eos and a Trojan mortal named Tithonus. Eos's desire for immortality for her human lover was acknowledged by the gods and Tithonus joined the immortals. Unfortunately, the goddess neglected to request that the man retain his youth. Consequently, Tithonus was doomed to continue to age forever until, having acquired all the infirmities of old age including senility, he was confined eternally to a dark dungeon. The lesson is clear: there is nothing to be desired in longer life, if the quality of that life is severely diminished.

Should it become possible to extend life expectancy to 120 years, as some have suggested, it will be necessary to extend the years of productive labor, to accompany a guarantee of longer life with a guarantee of longer years of good health, and to find ways to keep population growth in check. Perhaps science fiction visionaries like Isaac Asimov have the answer: humans will begin to populate outer space and perhaps end up overpopulating it too! (See Asimov's wonderful tale "The Deep.")

LIFE IS BRIEF, THE TIME IS SHORT

It is interesting to discover that the ancients had realists just as we do. Despite the fiction, they knew that life was brief, so they urged that it should be enjoyed now. At Egyptian banquets, a blind harpist would sing to remind guests that it was decreed

> That the bodies of men shall pass away and disappear
> And that others shall come to succeed them.

He sang of past heroes whose crumbled and forgotten tombs testified to the temporal nature of fame. The harpist was skeptical of beliefs in the afterlife because

> No one returns from where they are
> To describe their condition,

> To tell us of their surroundings.
> Or to comfort our hearts,
> Or to guide us to the place where they have gone.

In view of the ignorance of afterlife, he advised living life to the full in present time.

> So anoint your head with perfumed oils,
> Dress in exquisite garments,
> Scent your body with precious perfumes
> Which are the gifts of the gods,
> Occupy yourself with pleasure day by day,
> And don't stop seeking enjoyment for yourself.

He ended his song with this counsel:

> The best thing for you to do is to
> Seek to fulfill your heart's desire so long as you live.
>   (Larue 1985)

Similar advice was given by Qoheleth, the teacher in Ecclesiastes who instructed his pupils to

> Go, then, eat your bread cheerfully, and drink your wine with an untroubled heart (mind); for God has already approved of what you do. Let your garments always be white (festive); and let there be no lack of oil for your head. Enjoy life with the woman you love, all the days of your meaningless life that God grants you under the sun, for that is your remuneration in life as you live and toil under the sun. Whatever your hand finds to do, do it with your might; for there is no doing or thought or knowledge or wisdom in Sheol (the grave), to which you are going. (Eccles. 9:7–10)

No great change in attitude toward longevity has occurred over the millennia. There has been a sharp rise in the number of elders living to "a ripe old age" in the twentieth century, and many of the prevalent attitudes reflect those of ancient times. There are still those who look to magical formulas to retard graying and wrinkles. Some continue the fruitless search for immortality—now through the claims of cryonics where hopes are raised for resuscitation of frozen corpses in some distant future. Some seek to fill their lives with action, joy, and happiness believing that it is better to burn out than rust out.

There is nothing particularly right or wrong with the desire for longevity. For some, a long life can be exciting and fruitful. For example, Claire of Quincy, California, who was born in 1885, is far more active socially and much more independent than many men and women far younger than she. She keeps the books for a senior citizen nutrition program, works in her garden, and attends meetings. In Cambridge, Massachusetts, at The Intergenerational Day Care Center at the Stride Rite Shoe Corporation, elders meet with preschoolers in a setting that provides care for both by involving the elderly in the activities and education of children. Elders who are active and involved appear to be healthier and happier than those who are not, and these elders enjoy longevity after the manner suggested by the Egyptian harpist and Qoheleth. To such lively elders, death can be viewed as a reality to be delayed as long as possible.

THE BENEFITS OF LONG LIFE

Developmental psychologists tell us that all humans pass through a series of stages before arriving at mature, integrated, self-actualization. Perhaps there are some who can become self-actualized at an early age but, for most of us, time is a key ingredient. In other words, longevity provides the time needed for the full ripening of the personality.

Longevity also provides the time necessary for individuals to connect with the past, appreciate the present, and contemplate the future. To youngsters, age thirty signifies old age; for those who are thirty years old the notion is nonsense. They do not feel old, act old, or look old, and they do not fit the popular stereotype of age. The elder can recognize stereotypes as a way of thinking that may function to deny efforts at vibrant living. Stereotypes lock in individuals and deny the wonderful potentials and variations that can be observed in any age group. Of course, some elders engage in their own brand of stereotypical thinking. Such persons can be recognized by their bigotry, their racism, their sexist attitudes, and their mockery of younger persons. But those elders who can appraise the whole of life, who have moved beyond restrictive and limiting ways of looking at life—who are open to new experiences and to the appreciation of the richness to be found in people of all ages, races, creeds, colors, sexes, roles, or occupations—these open-minded elders, are on a different track. They may feel sorry for those whose lives have remained restricted by narrow ways of thinking for many years. Dwarfed by conventions accepted in the early stages of life, they are unable to grow and blossom.

In other words, longevity provides the time needed by some to cultivate ethical and spiritual growth.

LONGEVITY AND WISDOM

A long life provides the time needed for the transformation of knowledge and experiences into wisdom. Of course not all elders are wise; some have been foolish and stupid throughout their lives and continue to be so in their old age. But there are others—and they are from all walks of life—who find time to reflect and develop a sense of the sum, substance, and the meaning of their lives. They ponder their life-journey and perhaps are able to transmit to others something of what they have learned. This is what the philosopher Socrates suggested when he visited the elderly Cephalus:

> There is nothing which for my part I like better, Cephalus, than conversing with aged men; for I regard them as travelers who have gone on a journey which I too may have to go, and of whom I ought to enquire, whether the way is smooth and easy, or rugged and difficult. (*The Republic,* I:328)

In those cases where longevity burdens individuals who suffer with physical and mental handicaps like those of Tithonus, long life can become an impossible affliction. It is a moving and unnerving experience to visit acute care wards in nursing homes where elders lie with mouths agape, fed by tubes, and kept alive by machines and drugs. The national commitment to life, liberty, and the pursuit of happiness can appear to have undergone a transition to become the prolongation of life, with confinement devoid of happiness—a modern version of the Tithonus story. In other words, the "right-to-life" slogan can be overextended to the point of becoming unethical. To argue, as some will, that God gave life and only God should take it away, can condemn a suffering individual to an existence marked by excruciating pain relieved only by drugs that stupify. Compassion and the right of the individual to choose death are set aside in favor of theology and, like Tithonus, the elder is imprisoned in a diminished quality-of-life environment. At this point, the validity of the claims of euthanasia must be faced (see chapter 19).

LIMITATIONS OF LONGEVITY

The limitations placed on the acquisition of a joyous and meaning-filled old age are primarily related to personal freedom, independence, health, and finances, but may also include family relationships. Many elders cope with the issues magnificently (see chapter 18); they move from the freedom of full independence to semidependence and even into complete dependency, and somehow seem to be able to maintain a high degree of independence of spirit. They accomplish this by always considering options, by always recognizing that there are choices to be made and that they can make these choices for themselves. As their health begins to change—for example, as the pain of arthritis increases—they make contingency plans to maintain personal control even though their choices may be limited.

Some older adults express control over their lives by determining to age at home. They become part of the 95 percent of elders who eschew nursing homes and long-term care facilities. Not all are in good health, and many rely on home health care services and adult day care. But they are in their own homes, with their own familiar surroundings, in a neighborhood they know and understand. They may depend on their families for assistance with medical care, housekeeping, shopping, transportation and so on, but they are on familiar turf.

After the death of her husband, one seventy-year-old woman who had never learned to drive gave the family car to her son and daughter-in-law who lived nearby, with the proviso that the daughter-in-law drive her to her doctor's office for appointments, to the drug store for medications, to the grocery store for food shopping, and so on. Neither the elder nor her son and daughter-in-law are wealthy, but they have worked out a balancing of costs that accommodates both families. The elder buys gasoline for the car; her son and daughter-in-law pay for auto maintenance. Their arrangement points up the fact that in most family caregiver situations, it is often the daughter or daughter-in-law who becomes the primary caregiver. Where family feelings are amicable, the burdens of responsibility can be handled without friction. On the other hand, when the daughter has responsibilities to a family as well as to the elder, the problems of the "sandwich generation" surface.

THE SANDWICH GENERATION

The term "sandwich generation" identifies the dilemma experienced by middle-aged children of elders. They are at a "stage" in life where, as they let go of their youth and cope with the responsibilities of raising adolescent children still living at home, they are confronted with aging parents needing attention and perhaps assistance and support. Social and personal "oughts" can place obligations for the care of aging parents onto middle-aged children, which are in opposition to the younger adults' desire for the unity and identity of their own households. Love for the parents who raised them can come into conflict with personal wishes for familial autonomy. Concern for the health and safety of older loved ones can induce the desire to rescue these elders. Conflicts can arise when families face financial and parenting pressures with teenaged children who are expressing their desire for independence and who want to pursue a college education. The result can be mixed feelings of guilt, helplessness, and frustration for both the elders and their children (Silverstone 1979, p. 108). Sometimes the burdens create tensions leading to abuse (see chapter 7).

The ethical issues involved are related to generally accepted notions of the obligations of children for their parents and what aging parents can expect (demand) of their children. In most societies, tradition, enhanced by religion, has taught that children are responsible for their aging parents and that parents have a right to expect care in their old age. For example, when I was in Hebron, Israel, in 1967 right after the six-day war, a young Arab businessman expressed his distaste for living under Israeli rule. He had his savings in Amman, Jordan, and his skills could easily have been transferred to Jordan. I suggested that he move. He was shocked. How could he abandon his ninety-year-old parents who were untroubled by the Israeli presence inasmuch as they had lived peaceably with Jews before the 1948 partition of Palestine? As the eldest son, the businessman had social and family obligations that simply could not be ignored. He could not have lived with himself had he moved even though he knew his aged parents were quite happy looking after themselves and their large fruit farm. What was equally important was that his parents and the society in which he lived *expected* him to be there for his elders.

Not every family lives with such powerful social controls, but the bonds of love and caring, and the feelings of "ought" cannot easily be ignored. In modern Western society population mobility adds to the problem. Many young families live hundreds or even thousands of miles from the parental home. In a new environment, the young families have adopted new living patterns. The elders may have maintained traditional values and modes of living, while the offspring may have accepted different values and more modern lifestyles. On the other hand, the young parents, both holding jobs, may have developed very regimented household practices for efficiency and the control of their children, while the elders may have become more relaxed and laid back as they contemplate the important dimensions of life that can be overlooked during the course of a busy schedule. They may contemplate existence in the manner of the following lines:

> If I had to live my life over I'd dare to make more mistakes next time. I'd relax, I would limber up, I would be sillier than I have been this trip. I would take fewer things seriously. I would take more chances. I would take more trips. I would climb more mountains, swim more rivers. I would eat more ice cream and less beans. I would perhaps have more actual troubles, but I'd have fewer imaginary ones.
>
> You see I'm one of those people who live seriously and sanely hour after hour, day after day. Oh, I've had my moments, and if I had to do it over again, I'd have more of them. In fact, I'd try to have nothing else. Just moments, one after another, instead of living so many years ahead of each day. I've been one of those persons who never goes anywhere without a thermometer, a hot water bottle, a raincoat, and a parachute. If I had to do it again, I would travel lighter than I have.
>
> If I had to live my life over, I would start barefoot earlier in the spring and stay that way later in the fall. I would go to more dances. I would ride more merry-go-rounds. I would pick more daisies. (anon.)

Such a relaxed lifestyle may not be acceptable or available to a harried couple in the sandwich generation. The ideas might sound wonderful but their lives are so structured that any attempt to introduce such thinking into the family setting could only be seen as destructive and disrupting. Of course not all elders are so laid back and carefree; many continue the restrictive, up-tight life patterns regretted in the statement, and such a rule-bound and rigid approach can be equally troublesome to the harried sandwich generation.

When two different life patterns are compressed into one household, friction is bound to occur before harmonious arrangements can be achieved. Sometimes yielding to another's wishes and giving up cherished attitudes can produce inner stress. On the other hand, there are families that have been able to integrate a three- and even a four-generation household successfully.

In actuality, there is no rule that children *must* care for their elders.

In families where relationships are strained, the very idea is recognized as unproductive and unhealthy. Where strong bonding patterns exist, where caring people are involved, where personal and social conscience suggest responsibility, both parents and children can expect that if and when elders are in need, their children will be on hand to help. Whereas in the past, the responsibility for elder care could be shared among several children, today because of smaller families the burden of responsibility falls on a few. In most cases, the daughter becomes the responsible child and the daughter's family becomes "the sandwich generation."

WITHOUT THE SANDWICH

For needy elders who do not have family support, society bears the responsibility for aid. Within the confusing maze of community based services, the elderly can find help to deal with everything from shopping to meal preparation, from yard work to transportation. Some, who cannot cook for themselves, rely on meals-on-wheels or attend local synagogue, church, or community centers where food is served. Many communities provide transportation that enables the handicapped elder to meet medical appointments.

LONGEVITY AND HEALTH

Perhaps the most important contribution to a meaning-filled long life is good health. To be old, frail, in poor health, aching in every bone and muscle, confined to a bed or wheelchair, spending the greatest part of the day and night in sleep or drowsy semi-awareness is hardly an encouraging advertisement for longevity. Heroic health-care measures that keep the fragile old alive in a semi-comatose state, with only fragmentary awareness of the world about them, are simply unethical. Life-saving has become more important than health-saving.

We are total human beings, not simply biological objects. "A sound mind in a sound body" marks the healthy person. But mind and body, spirit and feeling, relationships and environment, dreams and aspirations, memories and meaning contribute to the whole person. We may suffer small or partial limitations in either mind or body and still be fulfilled human beings. When the other dimensions of the personality decay and the individual is reduced to a helpless, breathing shell of the self, longevity is no longer to be desired, and continuing existence can be recognized as an evil.

At this point, some theologians will demur arguing that every life is precious to God no matter what state the person may be in. One should, therefore, accept the wonderful benefits of modern medicine and appreciate longevity as a symbol of divine blessing, just as it was accepted in biblical times. Some medical practitioners may also protest, arguing that they interpret their calling as a commitment to preserve life, to fight disease, and to prolong life as much as possible. To each of these I can only say that there comes a time when theology and blind commitment to a philosophy can be challenged by reality. For me and for others like me, love takes precedence over existence, and quality of existence over longevity. My love of others and of life itself makes longevity desirable only if and when the quality of life can still be part of being. If, like Abraham, an elder can find some one to love (Keturah) and has still the vigor to produce children, then one can hail the wonders of whatever modern medicine can do to make such an existence possible. On the other hand, the quality of Tithonus's long life symbolizes the meaninglessness of such a life without quality. To strive to live only to achieve Tithonus's kind of longevity is unethical. As the number of elders increases, it is clear that if ethical concerns do not prompt responses to the problems of longevity, then economic factors will.

Not much can be done to alter the course of life for those who are presently old. A healthy old age is possible for the future if the steps discussed in the upcoming chapter on health (chapter 14) are initiated now. Hope for a healthy longevity begins at birth. One can predict only trouble and perhaps a short life for the hundreds of babies born addicted to drugs because their parents were addicts. If modern parents are educated to think of the health and lives of their children in terms of longevity, the life-enhancing patterns they initiate now can give promise of a healthy longevity for the future.

REFERENCES

Bryan, Cyril P. 1974. *Ancient Egyptian Medicine: The Papyrus Ebers.* Chicago: Ares Publishers, Inc. (reprint of 1930 edition).

Gaster, Theodor H. 1976. *The Dead Sea Scriptures.* New York: Anchor Books.

Johnson, Horton A., ed. 1985. *Relations Between Normal Aging and Disease.* New York: Raven Press.

Jowett, B., trans. 1937. *The Dialogues of Plato*. New York: Random House, vol. 1.

Larue, Gerald A. 1985. "Historical Perspectives on the Role of the Elderly," in Gari Lesnoff-Caravaglia, ed., *Values, Ethics and Aging*. New York: Human Sciences Press, pp. 41–55.

———. 1988. *Ancient Myth and Modern Life*. Long Beach, Calif: Centerline Press.

Leonard, Jon L., J. L. Hofer, and N. Pritikin. 1976. *Live Longer Now*. New York: Charter Books.

Pelletier, Kenneth R. 1982. *Longevity: Fulfilling our Biological Potential*. New York: Dell Publishing Co.

Pepper, Claude. 1979. *Americans over 100*, U.S. House of Representatives. Washington, D.C.: Government Printing Office. Committee Publication, #96-203, November 14.

Roan, Shari. 1990. "Researchers Try to Raise Quality of Extended Life," *The Los Angeles Times*, March 27.

Silverstone, Barbara. 1979. "Issues for the Middle Generation: Responsibility, Adjustment, and Growth," in Pauline K. Ragan, ed., *Aging Parents*. Los Angeles: University of Southern California Press, pp. 107–15.

Stanford, Barbara. 1983. *Long Life and Happiness*. Santa Monica, Calif.: Long Life Center.

Vermes, G. 1973. *The Dead Sea Scrolls in English*. Baltimore, Md.: Penguin Books.

Vreeland, Leslie. 1990. "The Drug of the Decade?" *Ladies Home Journal*, October, pp. 91–92.

12

Fear and Aging

"Competence in old age is inevitably subject to comparison with competence at earlier ages."

—Erikson, Erikson, and Kivnick, *Vital Involvement in Old Age,* p. 165

For some, perhaps for many, there is something rather scary about aging. In part, the fear grows out of awareness of the development of limitations. We can no longer leap over fences as we once could. We step down from a chair carefully, rather than hopping down as we did some years ago. We become aware of the loss of physical potentials and fear the loss of more. For the younger person, watching these restrictions on actions and activities in others can produce uneasiness and a fear of aging.

For the elder, fear of consequences caused by exceeding one's ability to perform can be beneficial. News reports broadcast that when Carroll O'Connor was to be welcomed into the Television Hall of Fame, he was confronted with a choice. He could attend the ceremonies by flying from Florida to Hollywood, then back again, or he could accept the honor by appearing on remote television. He chose not to attend. He was recovering from a recent operation and decided to protect his health by remaining in Florida. O'Connor could have chosen to make the trip and no doubt there was an earlier time in his life when the fact that he was recovering from an operation would not have prevented him from attending this public recognition of his acting. But he is older now and age has placed limits on what he can and should do. He wisely chose to protect his health. Fear or concern for doing harm to his body guided his response.

147

My brother-in-law Bob was always a do-it-yourselfer. He climbed the ladder to trim the trees and change the storm windows. Suddenly, when he was in his late sixties, he felt insecure on the ladder. He was afraid he might fall. He decided he was too old to do these regular household chores. Age caused changes in his body and brought on feelings of instability and vulnerability in a setting that was familiar to him—feelings he had never before experienced. Bob's fear of falling and awareness of age-related loss of physical skills prompted him to choose not to test his desire to be in charge of all aspects of gardening or responding to seasonal changes, but to relax and let someone else do the work.

I watch her as she strides down the street for her brisk evening walk. Helene is sixty-eight and determined that she will not encounter the physical limitations she has seen in friends of her age. She is exercising so that she can move up to a level of physical fitness that will enable her to participate in five- and ten-kilometer runs. She has seen young people awed by elders who are her age as they line up for these runs, clad in the latest jogging outfits. The elders often outpace and outlast their younger competitors. Helene has a combined fear of aging in general and of what aging can do to a person; she is confronting those fears head-on with her best efforts to delay or deny the physical limitations associated with aging. She fights her fears with a positive life-enhancing program of exercise.

Far more discomforting than physical aging is the awareness of mental decay. Ethel was sixty years old when she was informed that she had the incurable Alzheimer's disease and that, over time, it would produce increasing mental impairment. She is still in the early stages and she and her husband, Rob, seem to handle their daily lives despite the disease. But Ethel is frustrated. She forgets all sorts of details and she draws blanks when trying to recollect recent activities, though she has always kept up with the news. Today Ethel may read a newspaper article, only to read it again because she cannot remember what she had just read. She misplaces things. She had been an accountant and office manager for a large company; today she can't balance a checkbook, or remember whether she paid bills or entered the payment in her records. Rob has taken over this responsibility. Little by little her confusion and her distress grow, too, over what is happening to her. And little by little Rob's concerns grow because Alzheimer's is not a one-person disease—it affects the caregiver as well as the victim.

Ethel is not alone. It is estimated that about four million Americans are afflicted with Alzheimer's. More than 50 percent of all nursing home patients have Alzheimer's and more than 47 percent of elders eighty-five years of age and older have the disease. It is estimated that the cost for care of Alzheimer's victims amounts to more than $80 billion per year, including diagnosis, treatment, nursing home care, informal care, and lost wages (Larson 1990).

How long does the illness last before the patient dies? The life span of Alzheimer's patients is anywhere from three to more than twenty years. It is not surprising to find that Alzheimer's disease is listed as the fourth leading cause of death among adults after heart disease, cancer, and stroke (Larson 1990).

What can be done for Alzheimer's victims? Nothing beyond giving care and love. There is, at present, no cure and no way of stopping the progress of the disease. Some families are able to care for the person at home, with family members taking shifts to look after the victim. In one case, the patient, a large, strong woman, would throw childish tantrums and because of her strength her violent outbursts threatened the security of the family. With some reluctance and some guilt but with genuine feelings of relief, the family found a nursing home where she could be cared for. They visit her regularly but the visits become more and more meaningless as her memory fades.

The fear engendered by this disease is threefold. First, the victim fears what is happening; second, the caregivers fear the development of the disease; and third, those who see their friends, companions, and relatives develop the symptoms of Alzheimer's begin to fear and worry about the possibility of acquiring the disease themselves as they age.

Of course, fading memory does not always indicate the onset of Alzheimer's. Vascular dementia or multi-infarct disease, resulting from a series of mini-strokes in the small arteries of the brain, probably due to hypertension or high blood pressure, can damage brain tissue. Malnutrition, thyroid problems, use of alcohol, and even infections can produce symptoms that could be mistaken for Alzheimer's. Wrong dosages of drugs and medications or the mixture of certain drugs and medications can cause physical and mental reactions. Moreover, when elders are depressed, anxious, bored, or lonely, or with lowered self-esteem, they may become disoriented and exhibit memory losses that parallel dementia. Of course, these situations can be remedied. What is most important is that before memory loss is labelled Alzheimer's disease, careful, accurate, and proper diagnosis by a qualified physician be undertaken.

COPING WITH DISABILITIES

What are the ethical responses to physical and mental losses associated with aging? First, it is important to recognize that a minority of elders are really troubled by these infirmities. Only 5 percent of elders over sixty-five years of age are in institutions, and while this statistic involves a huge number of people, it is comforting and exciting to know that most elders live among us on their own or with their families.

Second, despite the physical limitations that come with age, some 80 percent of elders have no real limitations on their mobility. Most are well and are willing to recognize and confront the fears that can accompany the awareness of limitations imposed by age. For many elders, the fear is replaced by a realism that asserts that "this is the way it is and one learns to flow with the tide of change." Froim Camenir put it this way:

> My daily routine as an 83-year-old man (except for a change in the quantity of physical work) is no different from when I was age 73, or 63, or 53. It is true that, physically, the body becomes weaker, and we cannot perform the work or activities that we could in our younger days. (Camenir 1978, p. 172)

Third, the love and care of others for the victim of fear are the most responsible reactions. The development of a nourishing environment encourages the victim to recognize growing infirmities as part of the aging process and to fight back insofar as it is possible by exercising the body, watching diet, doing chores that can be done without worrying. If the infirmity is mental, then by engaging in conversations that help to keep the mind active, by exercise and careful diet the quality of life, no matter how severely limited, is maximized.

Fourth, therapy and peer-group counseling can be helpful. Victims and caregivers learn from others how to deal effectively with their problems. In extreme cases where patients are deeply troubled and disturbed, medications including tranquilizers or antidepressants may be called for to ease the fears and tensions. It is very important that social support for the family of the victim be available.

REFERENCES

Camenir, Froim. 1978. "How an Eighty-Three-Year-Old Man Looks at Life," in *The New Old: Struggling for Decent Aging.* Garden City, N.Y.: Anchor Press, pp. 172–74.

Erikson, Erik H., Joan M. Erikson, and Helen Q. Kivnick. 1986. *Vital Involvement in Old Age.* New York: W. W. Norton & Company.

Freedman, Gail A. 1985. "Age and Memory Loss: Myth and Reality," *Family Circle,* February 26, pp. 71–77.

Larsen, David. 1990. "Future of Fear," *The Los Angeles Times,* March 18, pp. E1, E8.

13

Elder Care, Elder Love

"Society's reality differs from love's reality. The strength to believe in love when you are pitted against a nonreinforcing proving ground is more than most people can accept. So they find it easier to put love aside, to reserve it for special people on unique occasions and join forces with society in questioning its supposed reality.

"To be open to love, to trust and believe in love, to be hopeful in love and live in love, you need the greatest strength."

—Leo Buscaglia, *Love,* pp. 192–93

QUESTION: Why do you want to work in Gerontology?
ANSWER: Well, in the first place, I just love old people . . .

The answer is positive, affirmative, acceptable, but it is also naive. To begin, all elders are not lovable. Some may be, but others can be crotchety, belligerent, bigoted, cruel, and vindictive—just like those who are younger. Old age does not automatically produce a lovable character; individuals carry into old age most of the qualities they exhibited during their lifetime. Some changes may occur. A rather strict parent may become a relaxed and permissive grandparent. A tight-fisted, hard-nosed business person may become a generous and open-handed retiree. But it is important to recognize that elders are just people and they represent the manifold dimensions of character, attitudes, and personality that can be found in every community or assemblage of persons. Love is important, but professionals who work with and live with elders must be aware of the problems, responsibilities, and even dangers of open love and learn where boundaries must be set.

Love signifies affirmation. It testifies to worth. It expresses belonging and caring. To love and to care is to become a caregiver. Such love is, perhaps, the supreme ethical quality for life. Without love, persons are isolated, alone, and barred from intimacy with others. Without love, individuals often feel unlovely, unlovable, and rejected, with such feelings producing dejection and depression.

I still carry within me the words of a seventy-year-old man: "I hate myself. I have always hated myself. I have no friends. Even my neighbors in the mobile home park where I live ignore me." To me, he came across as an intelligent, alert, capable, helpful, caring individual. He was easy to talk with—a bit tense perhaps, but eager and willing to share and listen. Apparently, what I perceived was just the shell, the outer appearance. Inside was a hurting, lonely, unloved, and angry person. The conversation came after I had given a lecture on the search for meaning in life. There was no chance to probe the background or reasons for his self-hatred in this public setting. How terrible must be his inner pain and how deep his longing for acceptance!

THE NEED FOR BOUNDARIES

Elders who are isolated from family and placed in nursing homes find their basic survival needs met by persons who, no matter how warm and concerned they may be in their professional roles, are members of another family with ties outside the institution. Caring persons who become professionals are (or should be) taught, trained, and warned not to become emotionally involved with patients. Emotional attachment by the caregiver not only violates the standard code of ethics governing professional-client relationships, but tends to threaten the validity and efficacy of the relationship. This is not to suggest that caregivers should become cold, unfeeling, businesslike automatons; care by such persons would reduce the relationship to nothing more than a mechanical fulfilling of the patient's basic needs. Care involves acting for the elder's well-being. Of course, there will be transference, just as there is in any clinical setting. One cannot touch and physically assist an elder without producing some aspects of bonding.

To care means to become involved. How much involvement can busy ward aides, social workers, nurses, doctors, resident managers, and others handle? One medical doctor developed a daily habit of greeting each nursing home resident when he first entered the building and walked down the halls. He would pause briefly, speak to each person and perhaps comment on the way they looked or refer to some person or event that had meaning for the individual. Later, when he might be deeply preoccupied with a health problem, he would pass by residents whom he had greeted earlier without paying much attention to them. Some expressed hurt at being ignored. Some felt that they must have done or said something to offend him. Others felt that he must have gotten into trouble. And so on. The bonding was more effective than he had imagined possible. Some residents felt that he had an obligation to recognize them *every* time he passed by—a duty that could become burdensome.

He was not the doctor who breezed through the institution, handing out prescriptions with little or no examination, spending the minimum amount of time listening with impatience to a resident's litany of ailments. He was not "Dr. Cheerful" who tended to dismiss patient complaints with a wise crack, "You are probably tiring yourself fighting off the ladies in this place, Mr. Brown!" He was the doctor who took blood pressure three times—once when they were sitting, once when they stood, and again after they had walked a bit. He was the one who paid attention to their gait, to their balance. He was the caregiver who gave care. And the residents knew how fortunate they were to be in a nursing home where he was the doctor. But some forgot that no single person could demand all of his time or attention and that he was under no obligation of love and care to give individuals his attention *every* time he passed by.

Medical persons—doctors, dentists, nurses, therapists, and others—are elevated to special status in nursing homes. In good, well-run settings, they have time for their patients, they care about them, and they feed the patient's need for recognition. These professionals know that patients are sensitive and that slighting an individual can lower self-esteem and cause inner hurt. They are committed to something more than merely treating the patient's latest ache or pain. They seek to help patients rehabilitate themselves. The medical staff encourages the development of an environment that promotes good health. They do all of this because they care about their profession, they care about themselves as caregivers, and they care about their patients. As caregivers of status, these professionals must set and maintain boundaries that maximize their effectiveness without taking anything away from their expressions of caring.

The importance of setting boundaries is not limited to nursing homes. A caring family learned that a lonely elderly widow who lived nearby had contemplated suicide because she felt no one cared. They invited her for an outing and to their home for Sunday dinner. Soon the woman was there every Sunday. Next, it became clear that she expected to go with the family on other outings. She visited often during the week, just before meal time so that she was invited to dine with the family. Often she stayed late into the evening, watching television and encouraging others to listen to her favorite programs. She began to interfere in the raising of the children. In the words of the children, "She was a drag." How does one break overbonding without completely rejecting the person? More important: How does one set limits on caring for persons who are not part of one's intimate circle?

Boundaries must be established at the outset and the easiest way to do this is by introducing formalities that imply limits. The staff in a nursing home, or the neighbor, can always be addressed as Mr. or Mrs. so-and-so, not as (good old) Charlie or (dear) Susie. The lonely widow does not become "aunt" to the children. In return, the elder learns to address the caregiver in the same formal terms. Language provides the barrier to an intimacy that is not essential to caring. Such formalities, when universally practiced, avoid the debasing paternalism implicit in situations where residents address caregivers in the institution formally but are, in turn, addressed informally.

When residents (or neighbors) begin to pry into the personal life of caregivers by seemingly innocuous questions, it is important to say, "I never bring my personal life into the residence," or "We are a very private family and while we are pleased to invite you for dinner once in a while, we know you will respect our privacy as we respect yours." Does this seem cold and unfeeling? Perhaps it does. On the other hand, it issues a demand for respect. It sets limits on relationships. It is far more reasonable and respectful than the bland "I must love everyone" approach, which opens doors that may be difficult to close. It acknowledges that "I don't want everyone in my private circle and I do not want others to become overdependent on me."

THE FAMILY AND THE NURSING HOME

The greatest problems produced by the love-bond are in the family, and the burdens most often fall on women. As we have noted, modern women are entering the work force in numbers unprecedented in history. Nevertheless, when the elder declines to a stage where help is needed, the care responsibilities usually become the lot of the daughter or, less often, the daughter-in-law. In such settings, feelings of affection can become strained. A dependent elder whose dependency is at the level of a child does not call forth the feelings of willing and eager response associated with a child's needs. The child will grow beyond its present requirements; the elder sinks deeper into dependency. Sometimes the burden becomes too great for both the prime caregiver and the family, and the elder is placed in a nursing home.

Placing an elder in a nursing home can become a trying test of love. Older family members may feel that they are being rejected, cast out, and no longer loved. Their tears and cries of pain can tear at the heart. The family feels guilt and perhaps a sense of failure. Somehow they ought to have been able to keep their elder at home. In reality, the responsibility for home care was beyond their ability, the greater act of love was to place the elder where adequate and proper care was available.

A caring family makes sure that the elder is placed in a well-run establishment. The nursing home should be visited without an appointment; only then is it possible to see the institution in its everyday setting. The smell and look of a nursing home can convey a lot—the odor of staleness or urine, and a dreary atmosphere become warning signs. The activity of the staff, whether focused on their own interests as they chat at the entry desk or on the patients as they work with them, suggests the kind of care available. Of course the family will check on the reputation of the institution and will inquire about what facilities are available for medical care, for recreation, for expression of interests, for the receiving of visitors, and discover what ethical codes underlie the operation. Each of such inquiries is a statement of love and care. The ethic of familial love calls for efforts to seek the best facility and the most life-affirming environment for an elder who must be cared for in a nursing facility.

Loving care does not end with placement of the elder in the best care facility. An elder in a nursing home puts new and continuing claims on the energies and time of family members and friends. Time must be scheduled for the visits that affirm, visibly and clearly, that love and caring are not diminished by change in locale. Often, it is assumed that because elders are in nursing homes they are "being cared for" and thus family obligations are lessened. As visits become fewer in number, the elder may feel abandoned. If the elder was seriously ill in a hospital, visits would be a daily occurrence. Residence in a nursing home is perceived differently, even though the need for the reassurance of love in this setting is just as important. As Leo Buscaglia notes, love calls for "great strength" and one might add, unflagging commitment and awareness of the elder's need for continuing reaffirmation of that love. Fortunately, in many and perhaps in most families, elders are not abandoned when necessity calls for placement in nursing home facilities. Visits continue to be regular and often. Phone calls punctuate the time between visits. Elders are reassured that they continue to matter. The demands on familial time are considered inconsequential because feelings of love and caring are dominant.

SO, YOU WANT TO BE A GERONTOLOGIST

We now go back to the student who "loves" elders. The feelings are real. They may have been engendered through association with grandparents or with elders who contributed to the student's maturation, or they may have grown out of humanitarian and humanistic concern for elder well-being. No matter what the source, the feelings are genuine. I have found them in pre-med students who will become geriatricians, in dental students who will focus part of their skill in treating elder needs, in those who will become nurses, and among those who plan to manage care facilities.

In an age where the "me" generation is supposed to be dominant, the presence of so many young men and women with altruistic aims is indeed heartening. Their love of elders and their plan to commit their careers to caring for older adults does not negate their desire to earn a decent standard of living. What is indicated is that they prefer to earn their livelihood in work that is service oriented and directed toward the aged. It is important that they be aware that altruistic love can place heavy demands on the giver—demands of time, energy, and patience. Many of these dedicated young people are well aware of this reality for they have given of their time in various elder settings, including nursing homes, senior centers, Alzheimer care groups, and others. Most are realistic. Most have faced difficult elder environments. Nevertheless, they continue to be dedicated.

These are the young people who inspire hope for better treatment of elders in the future. As they commit themselves to their particular professional goals, they automatically become involved in changing the world of elders that they themselves will one day enter. Their dedicated love gives us hope for elder care that will continue to be supportive of aging persons and that will seek to maintain elder dignity and feelings of worth.

REFERENCES

Ball, Avis Jane. 1986. *Caring for an Aging Parent.* Buffalo, N.Y.: Prometheus Books.

Buscaglia, Leo. 1972. *Love.* New York: Fawcett, 1972.

Fox, Nancy. 1986. *You, Your Parent, and the Nursing Home.* Buffalo, N.Y.: Prometheus Books.

Gelfand, Donald E. 1984. *The Aging Network: Programs and Services.* New York: Springer Publishing Company.

Karr, Katherine L. 1991. *Promises to Keep: The Family's Role in Nursing Home Care.* Buffalo, N.Y.: Prometheus Books.

14

Geroethics and Health

"Damn! Damn! Damn! Son of a bitch!"

—JoAnne

To mature, to age, is to experience change—physically, emotionally, mentally, and spiritually. Not all changes are pleasant. Some persons remain robust and hearty throughout life, suffering few ailments and little pain. The lives of others are afflicted by a variety of illnesses and deteriorating health. Obviously, it is preferable to be counted among those who enjoy good health, and it is clear that many elders work hard at maintaining soundness of body and mind. They exercise, watch their diet, avoid exposure to polluted air, are active in positive and worthwhile social activities, and focus their minds on issues and subjects that both challenge and stimulate them. Indeed, they are among those who expect, and are determined, to remain healthy until the day they die.

The majority of elders are relatively healthy until just before death. Then, suddenly, some seem to have one damaging experience after another. An elder will fall and break a hip, which requires hospitalization. During the period of limited and restricted activity the person appears to decline and become frail. Another older person, who has been active in life, suddenly contracts a bacterial infection. With JoAnne it was staphylococci in the spine that hospitalized her. As the medical team fought the infection, she suffered a heart attack and then two strokes. This active, involved, and much-loved woman now found herself trapped in a failing body. Her mind was as keen as ever but her speech came with difficulty due to a tracheal infection. She was not given to profanity, but one day, as her husband sat by her hospital bed, she looked down at her weakened and pain-filled body and expressed herself: "Damn! Damn! Damn! Son of a bitch!" When I heard the story, all I could think was: what an eloquent statement of frustration! She died after six months of continuing pain and misery.

Some of us—for example, the children of alcoholics or drug addicts—seem to be defeated from the outset. Their childhood is characterized by poverty, inadequate diet, depressing social settings, and often brutality. Some people have an inherited defective genetic trait (such as Huntington's chorea) that predetermines certain destructive health patterns. Others grow up without hope and without proper attention to health. Should they survive into old age, their existence is marked with inadequate treatment and suffering. In the United States the defeated often include poor, uninsured elders who depend solely on Medicare and Medicaid (the government health insurance program for the poor) for health protection. The costs of these programs have soared to billions more than annually projected—Medicare is currently $81.2 billion, up from $3.4 billion in 1986 (Dallek 1990). Consequently services have been reduced. Large corporations with health-care programs engage private screening organizations to weed out what is deemed to be unnecessary treatment while at the same time guaranteeing quality care. The emphasis everywhere seems to be on cutting back services.

To what extent is the individual, the family, and/or the government responsible for the maintenance of good health? This is the ethical issue that confronts society. If factors affecting good health extend from prenatal care to old age, what public social obligations are involved? During the past quarter century, laws have been passed that were designed to protect children, spouses, and elders from abuse (see chapter 7). It is obvious that society has concerns for physical, mental, financial, and spiritual well-being of the citizenry. Public welfare programs and community hospitals are further expressions of such concerns. How are elders involved?

THE NATIONAL HEALTH INSURANCE ISSUE

Caring families seek to do all they can for ailing elders, caring nations do the same. The inadequacy of health care in the United States raises moral and ethical questions that extend from individual treatment to social, economic, and medical policies. The fact that one of the wealthiest nations on the planet should be counted as one of two first-world countries (the other country is South Africa) failing to provide national health care for all its residents is nothing less than an obscenity. The records of inadequate treatment and debilitating costs that extend from cradle to grave, from newborns to elders, constitute an international medical scandal. Inferior prenatal health care places the United States twentieth in infant mortality among the twenty-two members of the Organization for Economic Co-operation and Development—thirteenth if African-American statistics are excluded (*Insight* 1988). Children suffering from treatable diseases die from lack of medical care because the costs are too high. For example, a seven-year-old died in Oregon in 1988 because it was decided that the limited Medicaid funds should not be spent for the bone marrow transplant that would have cost more than $100,000 (*Insight,* p. 12). Measles cases have risen from an average of about 3,000 per year from 1981 to 1988, to 26,000 with 97 potentially related deaths in 1990 because of low vaccination rates among the twelve million children living in poverty (Wielawski 1991). Elders needing home health care must be reduced to poverty before the Medicaid system steps in to help. Medical costs for doctors' fees and hospitalization are so excessive that families loose their assets and their spiritual nerve in attempting to care for ailing family members while trying to meet the costs of catastrophic illness. Where is the moral conscience in this great and powerful nation that enables it to tolerate these disturbing facts?

Despite the development of Health Maintenance Organizations (HMOs) and despite industrial health insurance programs, the costs to individuals and families continue to rise. To be sure, there is fat in the system that could be and should be eliminated. For example, overaggressive medical care inflates costs and some practitioners seem prepared to press their services to the limit of what the traffic will bear. Some have exploited both the system and elders by providing medical treatment that was not only unnecessary but dangerous to the aged patients so treated (Dean 1990). But other issues are involved as well. Inflation contributes to rising prices for health care. Developing medical technology renders equipment outmoded and the costs for new instruments can be astronomical, particularly when doctors and hospitals want the best and the latest for their patients. While it can be argued that American doctors rely too heavily on technology, it is also clear that as innovative technology becomes widespread, the cost of various frequent procedures are lowered and ultimately the healing process is enhanced.

The costs of seemingly endless miles of red tape involved in Medicare, Medicaid, HMOs, and insurance benefits continue to rise. Medical costs swell in keeping with the increasing number of litigations that require health providers to protect themselves with expensive insurance policies. Inflated health costs reduce the number of persons treated, which poses an ethical problem to citizens and their government.

Drugs are costly. Where generic drugs are available, elders can save tremendously by avoiding brand name medications. But some drug companies have patents that prohibit the production of generic counterparts. Drug company politics are not always honest; it is not unheard of for one company to seek to devalue the product of a competitor who offers medications that provide the same or better results. Doctors are not immune to the claims and pressures of drug advertisements; with a little well placed pressure, physicians can be persuaded to use the most expensive medications. Ultimately, it is the consumer, and in our case the elder, who has to pay the excessive prices. One cannot dismiss the fact that funds for research and development of new treatments are required, but drug companies are in a business that thrives on profits. While their products are important for human welfare; their procedures are often questionable.

What is the ethical response? Without question a national health insurance program that covers everyone is fundamental. For any American to be without health protection is immoral, and there is no reason why a national health program cannot be introduced. In the long run, health costs would be reduced through introducing prenatal care the effects of which would continue throughout the individual's life. Healthier babies grow up to be healthier adults. Healthy adults reduce the need for health care, and administrative costs would be dramatically reduced. Of course taxes would have to be increased, but who would object to paying more taxes for guaranteed health protection? Most of all, there would have to be a realignment of funds, reducing expenditures for destructive weaponry, chemicals, and machines and designating a greater percentage of national wealth for the welfare of the citizenry.

But, to be effective, a much broader and a more sane national health plan is required. For the government to be involved in a war against drugs while at the same time supporting a local narcotic industry (tobacco) is the height of folly. Further, the inconsistency of the government underwriting the cultivation, production, and merchandising of tobacco products while at the same time insisting that these products carry a surgeon general's warning about the health dangers of smoking is simply absurd. In Egypt, an intelligent businessman asked me, "Is it true that cigarettes in the United States carry a health warning from the surgeon general?" When I answered yes, he said, "I find that very amusing." I find it intellectually and morally insulting. What is even more disgusting is the knowledge that the products of this government-supported narcotic business are responsible for more than 400,000 deaths in America each year. One need only be with elders dying of smoking-induced lung cancer to become angrily aware of the unethical anti-health business in which the government is involved.

Quite rightly we express national concern for oil spills that foul the ocean waters and kill sea creatures; at the same time, we fail to protest the toxic wastes that spew from automobiles and affect the health of millions. Oil spills pale by comparison. Vehicles that can extend mileage per gallon or that run on low-cost and relatively nontoxic fuels are not put into production except experimentally. Only as air pollution reaches extremely dangerous proportions do oil companies seek to lower toxic emissions from gasolines, and only then do government officials and car manufacturers seek to reduce automobile emissions.

It has taken years for the government to initiate action designed to control the disposal of factory-produced industrial toxic wastes, and the coal smoke that results in acid rain, both of which affect life and health. For decades waste has been dumped in ravines then covered with landfill and later used for housing. Only when illness resulting from the seepage of dangerous chemicals from these landfills reaches epidemic proportions in area after area is any action taken. The government itself has been indifferent to the effects of military waste piles on communal health. For example, the largest producers of hazardous wastes in Orange County, California, are the Marine Corps air stations in Tustin and El Toro— two of the most polluted sites in the county (Johnson and Cone 1990). Once again, the question of the national ethic pertaining to health care comes to mind.

What can be done? Public health ethical issues involve choices. We, the people, can choose to continue in the same patterns or we can choose to pass legislation to safeguard individuals and communities. What is required is a broad national health policy. Such a policy would deny government support to producers of lethal drugs, such as tobacco. Indeed, advertising tobacco products, like advertising any other health threatening drug, should be forbidden. This same policy would regulate the disposal of waste products, with the government itself setting an example. Such a policy would emphasize recycling, the use of biodegradable packaging, reduction in the use of chemicals in agriculture and, in general, provide legislation aimed at health rather than profit only.

At the same time, while the national health program seeks to protect the general public, it must include education that places on every citizen the responsibility for exercise, diet, and regular health check-ups. How many elders were aware that the foods they were eating as young adults would ultimately contribute to their ill health? A friend who underwent multiple by-pass heart surgery commented that he had been raised on the rich Wisconsin meat, milk, and cheese diet with no awareness of the build up of cholesterol in his system until the heart attack occurred. He is not alone. Commercially packaged and canned foods are high in salts, sugars, and fats. Many bear deceptive labels such as "Lite" or "Low Cholesterol" without equal emphasis on the salt or sugar content. These products are consumed by elders and others who are not adequately informed about the relationship between food and health. We need responsible and accurate labeling of food products.

Of course, national health programs are not without problems. In Canada there are those who cannot find adequate words to praise the treatment received for illnesses that in the United States would have stripped the family not only of their financial reserves but their home as well. They point out that Canadian infant mortality is much lower than that of the United States (in 1981, 9.6 per thousand compared to 12.6 in the United States), that only 9 percent of the gross national product is spent on health care as compared to 12 percent in the United States. Most important, the burdensome, annoying, and counterproductive bureaucracy of the American system is reduced to a minimum in Canada. Where Canada falls behind is in the ready availability of the most advanced health care technology. For example, in the United States, hospitals demand their own magnetic resonance imaging equipment, lithotriptors to treat kidney stones, and so on. In Canada, the purchase of such equipment is limited by provincial budgets. Consequently, when the Ontario government paid over five million dollars to hospitals in Detroit to treat sick Canadians who could not receive immediate high-technology treatment in Canada, a question arose as to why that money had not been invested in Canadian hospital equipment or used to build a special unit for heart patients in Ontario (Walsh 1990).

It is pertinent to ask whether national health-care insurance will embrace the total needs of elders. For example, it is estimated that the two million people with Alzheimer's disease today could increase to eleven million by the year 2040. Whereas elders account for about 36 percent of national health expenditures today, that number could grow to 56 percent by 2040. At the same time, nursing home beds could outnumber hospital beds ten to one (Roan 1990).

The wealthy will always be able to buy the very best treatment, even when to do so would fly in the face of reason. For example, when the wealthy family of an eighty-four-year-old woman insisted that she be scheduled for a coronary bypass procedure despite medical advice that she could not possibly recover (she didn't), the doctor complied out of fear that he would be served with a lawsuit for failing to provide the best medical treatment. Such privileged mistreatment and waste of medical time and energy would still be possible for the wealthy under a national program, but not for the average citizen.

Another different problem lurks in the wings, but under the right set of circumstances it could move to center stage. When resources become scarce and costs soar, a national health policy could quietly come into being, one that limits treatment to persons falling within certain age groups, thereby providing elders with minimal care. This idea is related to triage.

TRIAGE

The word "triage" comes from a root meaning "to sift" or "to separate out." It has been used in times of national disaster or on battle fields to refer to the selection of patients for treatment, concentrating on those with potential for recovery and ignoring those whose situation is hopeless. Triage exists where demand for life-saving equipment and resources exceeds the supply. In wartime, the problems can be clearly defined. Patients are divided into three categories depending upon (a) the degree of need for immediate treatment, thus dressing a broken leg could be delayed in favor of attending to a hemorrhaging artery; (b) the amount of resources required, so that if the choice was between two wounded men, one requiring immediate extensive surgery to save his life and the other requiring less demanding surgery, preference would be given to the second person; and (c) the immediate future utility after treatment, so that a wounded soldier who could be patched up and returned to duty would be given preference over one whose needs would forgo a return to service. Here, time, resources, and utility are paramount considerations. Depending on the setting, other priorities could prevail.

In a nonmilitary setting, priorities for medical treatment often need to be established. For example, the semi-permanent shunt developed by Dr. Belding Scribner in the 1960s enabled patients to undergo repeated hemodialysis treatments without undergoing a succession of surgeries. But for more than a decade, until shunts became abundant, the shortage plagued dialysis programs and only a small fraction of patients whose lives could have been saved received treatment (Winslow 1982, pp. 12f). How are recipients selected under such circumstances? Would age be a consideration?

One can imagine a situation in which the choice to treat would be between a forty-year-old husband and father of two children and a sixty-eight-year-old retired elder and a grandfather, who lived with his wife. On what basis would the decision be made—age and estimated longevity, potential contributions to society, familial responsibilities, or maybe income? In a situation that did not demand immediate response, one can imagine a hospital ethics committee wrestling with the problem. But suppose the situation was complicated by funding for care issues and suppose a subtly agreed upon but undisclosed age limit had been established by medical authorities; then other considerations (except, perhaps, for the ability to pay) might be unimportant. Medical treatment could be denied simply on the basis of age. It is possible, and it may even be practical, to discriminate on the basis of age alone, and at that point national ideals of equality would become meaningless.

A form of triage is presently employed in County-USC Medical Center in Los Angeles. Due to a $7.6 million reduction in the County health care budget, the hospital, whose share was $4.2 million, introduced tougher criteria for treating patients, many of whom are poor, without medical insurance, and simply come without appointments to the walk-in clinic. As a result, approximately one in five persons are denied treatment. Only those with symptoms that could escalate into life-threatening or debilitating illness within a day or two receive care. Interestingly enough, here triage on the basis of age is not employed. Persons are not rejected simply because they are old. Dr. Richard May, one of the screening physicians, stated, "I don't turn elderly, frail people away. . . . Some of them are so confused I know they will never get to a health center if we don't take care of them here" (Wielawski 1990). Other local facilities have also been affected by the budget reduction and have cut back on adult out-patient services that will affect poor, sick people. In Los Angeles, triage is in operation, due to cutbacks in funding.

Moody (1985) reports that "the British system routinely rejects patients on grounds of age for certain medical procedures" (p. 43). Obviously, an age bias is already present; some persons are no longer deemed deserving of equal treatment. In all fairness, it must be admitted that Britain has far more home health care and spends far less on health services than the United States, yet enjoys a comparable life-span for its citizens (Moody 1985, p. 44). With the mounting costs of medical care for the aged in the United States, the developing of age-determined cutoffs for medical care may be on the horizon. Nevertheless, it must be remembered that the extension of life is as important for an elder as it is for a younger person. Nor is the "fairness" argument relevant: it reasons that because elders have already had a long life, medical attention should focus on those whose life trajectory offers more years than that of the elderly so that they, too, may enjoy an extended life. In those instances where an elder may choose not to undergo treatment, there is no problem: the elder is in charge of his or her own life and makes a personal choice. Neither decisions nor choices are made for the elder.

How can triage decisions be made fairly? Where the problem arises from shortage of resources and the candidates for treatment have approximately equal chances of recovery, the choice can be made according to random selection with no attention being paid to age, or on a first-come-first-served basis. Additional factors that might further refine the selection pool have included past, present, and future service to society, and familial responsibilities. In other words, age alone should not be the basis for denying treatment.

There can be little doubt that some aspects of triage will be introduced into medical programs as the aging population increases. The reasons for triage will be based on medical and treatment costs, availability of space and equipment, and on expenditures of professional time and energy. Where continuing or extensive medical treatment offers no hope of cure, only prolongs the dying process, and adds to the costs of mere existence, the hospice alternative can provide palliative care in terminal cases. Where there is hope of recovery and of an extended life of acceptable quality (acceptable, that is, to the elder) then agism should not interfere with the best medical care available.

ELDER HEALTH AND THE FAMILY

The family's response varies when faced with the sudden health problems of an elder relative. In some instances it is immediate: plans and priorities are set aside, while care for the ailing elder takes precedent over other concerns. The family reacts out of love and commitment. It is often stated that as the elder cared for the child, now the child reciprocates with care for the elder. When the illness requires long-term care and when the elder lives half a continent away, difficult decisions need to be made. How long can employment and family responsibilities be set aside? Should the elder be persuaded to move in with, or closer to, some family member? On the other hand, will occasional visits be enough to express feelings of love and responsibility? Distance has a dislocating effect on responses.

Other families may employ what has been called the "ostrich approach," a form of denial. The elder's emergency produces expressions of concern plus the argument that home and business responsibilities prohibit travelling or visiting or staying with the ailing person. Occasional letters and phone calls expressing concern, love, and regrets, or perhaps a short visit, serves to acknowledge awareness of the elder's situation, but both preclude involvement.

No one can decide for another what constitutes an appropriate response. Each family must weigh requirements for personal survival against feelings of what "ought" to be done. Failure to do what is expected by the elder, or what one's conscience suggests should be done, can produce guilt. Moving an elder to an unfamiliar area to be closer to the family can be upsetting to both the elder and the family in that it will engender new and immediate responsibilities for attention, entertainment, and care. There are no simple answers.

What is clear is that in view of the graying of America and of other nations, contingency plans need to be made. Families must discuss in advance what can be done in case of an emergency. Offspring can have at hand medical care data pertaining to their elder's health plans, medications, nearby hospitals, names and phone numbers of the elder's doctors, information about the elder's friends or neighbors, and so forth. What is most important is that the elder be part of and satisfied with the pre-planning. Most elders appreciate the sense of security that comes with knowing that the family is not only interested in their welfare but is willing to be involved.

When an emergency does occur, it is best if a single spokesperson represents the family, thereby avoiding an onslaught of questions and demands addressed to overworked hospital personnel and doctors. If out-of-town family members wish to be present at the time of an operation, a short initial stay with a follow-up visit when the elder is about to return home can be supportive and helpful, particularly if the elder lives alone. Most employers are willing to grant leave for family illnesses, and most families can manage to survive when one member is absent for a brief time. For the family, ethical responses can be practical, and practical responses can be ethical.

In some instances it is feasible to hire the services of private case managers, many of whom are trained social workers or nurses, to care for the needs of the recovering elder. Aging network services, state agencies on aging, senior centers, and church organizations can also become involved in responding to the needs of an ailing elder when the family lives far away and cannot be present. What is most important for the psychological health of the elder is the knowledge that the family cares enough to make an effort to help in time of crisis.

ELDER RESPONSIBILITY

Of all the characteristics of ailing elders, no matter what the origin of their illness, perhaps the most impressive is courage, closely followed by the ability to adapt (see chapter 18). Human existence is characterized both by dependency and interdependency. Our social patterns direct us toward employment to provide for the self and dependents. We like to feel that we have given in return for what we receive. "I earn my keep" is a familiar elder concept, which can be interpreted as "My work benefits others and at the same time earns money by which I can purchase what others have produced."

But there is another dimension of human life that moves beyond a businesslike *quid pro quo* arrangement, namely, the motivation to help and the desire to be helped (Skinner 1972, p. 283ff). Only as humans relate their individuality to their unity with others can the full human be actualized. Individuality in and of itself is important but it can also have little significance. The self is often validated largely through interaction with others.

The implications of interrelationship become apparent in the behavior of sick persons. Like those who are healthy, the ailing individual requires validation of continuing worth through the help of others, through the outreach of others, through the caring of others, through the touch of others. What is most important is that the relationship be genuine. Nothing is more destructive to feelings of self-worth than to sense that the treatment received in a nursing home or hospital setting is pro forma or robotlike and exercised without genuine concern for the sick person. The patient is reduced to something less than human, and is, perhaps, identified among members of the hospital staff as "the liver case" or "the old man" or "the old woman."

But elders must become involved in their own health care. It seems to me that the elderly have a moral responsibility to look after themselves and not simply depend on others to care for them. If they have developed poor health habits, changes can and should be made. Smokers can kick the habit. Much of the damage done by smoking can be repaired. In fact, within months of stopping the cigarette habit the functions of the heart and blood vessels begin to improve, despite the fact that the person has smoked for years. Within a year the former smoker's risk of a heart attack is virtually eliminated. Diets, too, can be changed. Menus that emphasize vegetables and cereal products, reduced sugar and salt can be tasty and healthy. Moderate exercise, such as walking, can be started. Elders can help themselves to better health and longer lives. Indeed, if they are prepared to look to others for assistance with health problems, they have the moral responsibility to act on their own behalf to benefit and if possible improve their own health. It is not fair or ethical to place the responsibilities for one's health solely on others.

DRUGS AND THE ELDERLY

Drugs may be defined as "any chemical substance that alters the function of one or more body organs or changes the process of a disease. Drugs include prescribed medicines, over-the-counter remedies, and the recreational, social and illicit use of drugs such as cocaine. Many foods and drinks contain small quantities of substances classed as drugs—tea, coffee, and cola drinks, for example, all contain *caffeine,* which is both a *stimulant* and a *diuretic drug.*" (*The A.M.A. Home Medical Encyclopedia,* Vol 1, 1989, p. 376). To this inclusive definition, one might add alcohol.

Although some elders may use cocaine, marijuana, or other illicit drugs for pleasure or relaxation or because of addiction, our focus will be primarily on prescribed medicines and over-the-counter remedies. As Edward S. Brady has noted, "No one can deny the need and value of medication in the lives of the elderly. Drugs can ease pain, halt infections, offset physiological changes, reduce anxiety and bring sleep." He goes on to say that when drugs are misused they can "stupify, injure, and generate serious problems" (1978).

The effects of drugs on elders is still under study. Some physicians prescribe for the aged as they do for younger patients. Melmon and Morelli warn, "The age of a patient, young or old, may change either the ability of the target organs to respond to drugs or the ability of normal systems to dispose of a drug or to oppose its effects" (1972, p. 551).

Drugs play an important part in treating psychological disorders in the aged which are sometimes viewed with "therapeutic pessimism"—an attitude which "is not justified," according to H. M. van Praag (1978, p. 423). He makes the following observation:

The automatic association of "old and disturbed" with "irreversible degeneration of brain tissue" is inappropriate, for two reasons: (a) elderly patients may suffer from "functional" psychological disorders, i.e., disorders in the aetiology of which degeneration of cerebral tissue is not an important factor or seems to have acted merely as a trigger; (b) organic cerebral damage in advanced age is not necessarily based on senile or arteriosclerotic processes and, moreover, can be reversible. (p. 423)

According to van Praag, "Drugs unequivocally able to delay or arrest the deterioration of neurons in the brain and the associated deterioration of intellectual functions are not available. We do, however, have drugs which are valuable in the treatment of: (a) psychiatric symptoms secondary to intellectual deterioration, and (b) psychiatric symptoms of senescence which do not seem to be directly related to the anatomical process of senescence" (p. 440). Because the studies of the brain and of human behavior are still being researched, "psychological disorders in the aged call for careful psychiatric and physical diagnosis" (p. 423).

Over many years of living, elders develop patterned ways of responding to pain. They have learned to use analgesics such as aspirin to reduce fever, treat joint pains, headaches, menstrual discomforts, and so on. They will have their own favorite brands of cough medicines and ointments and perhaps a collection of heating pads, inhalers, and vibrators. They may also indulge in family treatments such as lemon and honey for easing sore throats, oil of eucalyptus as a chest rub for colds, plus many more. In other words, most elders will have had a long history of treating the ordinary, everyday ailments and injuries that do not require professional intervention. They are accustomed to taking care of themselves.

It is when these ordinary household treatments no longer work, when an illness or a pain or some bodily dysfunction has moved beyond simple remedies, that medical intervention is required. Elders constitute only about 11 percent of the population, but they consume more that 25 percent of all drugs prescribed in this country. Beyond prescriptions, no one knows how many over-the-counter medications are used by elders.

The most common elder ailments requiring prescribed medication include heart conditions, high blood pressure, arthritis, mental and nervous disorders, gastrointestinal disorders, genito-urinary tract infections, diabetes, respiratory infections, circulatory infections, and chronic skin conditions (Lofholm 1978, pp. 11–17). When more than one of these conditions prevail, physicians and pharmacists must exercise extreme care in researching the possible effects of one prescribed medication on another and inform the elder of any possible consequences.

Most elders trust their doctors and their pharmacists and the prescriptions they provide. These older adults follow dosage regimens faithfully. Their prescriptions are filled regularly and with medical approval. They report back to their physicians any side effects. Then what is the problem? The problem lies with those who do not follow orders and whose use of medications tends to be erratic.

Some elders become overzealous in taking drugs. When prescriptions are changed they keep the remnants of a previous prescription, perhaps for years. Consequently some elders have cabinets cluttered with a variety of old and outdated medications. Some hate to waste expensive medicines, so they decide to use up the remaining dosages even as they begin taking the new. Others become so habituated to using a given drug that they continue having prescriptions refilled long after the need has passed. Still others forget to take their medication or forget that they have taken it and ingest a second dosage, and both underdosing and overdosing can have serious results. Some medications are time released and call for a regular regimen. When that regimen is violated problems can arise. Some elders may lack funds for expensive prescriptions and so put off buying needed drugs, while others take drugs that have not been prescribed and may have been purchased for use by someone else with what seems to be a similar ailment. If the elder has poor eyesight, dosages can be misread.

Doctors and pharmacists must learn not to assume that every elder understands the nature of prescribed medications. Many do not know why they are taking a certain drug. Where two drugs are prescribed for the treatment of different conditions, some elders may be confused as to which drug is designed for which ailment, and in instances where the daily dosages differ, the drugs may be inadvertently substituted in the elder's mind and wrong amounts taken. Often, tiny pills come in little bottles with print so small that it can only be read with a magnifying glass. Most persons have difficulty reading the fine print; for elders, the problem may be augmented by failing eyesight. The pharmacist may provide an advisory print-out on a separate piece of paper that would ordinarily be attached to a larger bottle; the instructions may be produced by a dot-matrix printer on paper that sometimes features a pharmacy logo as background (at least mine does). The information is hard to read and because it is not attached to the bottle it can be lost or discarded. Obviously, some doctors and some pharmacists have a lot to learn about elders, the ways in which they use prescriptions, and how they read or follow instructions.

Efforts to regulate use and misuse of drugs in nursing homes are still in process. Sedatives are used widely to control residents. It is reported that "overdosing and misuse of powerful psychoactive drugs are common in nursing homes across the nation, provoking terrible side effects and doing little to improve behavior" (Spiegel 1991, p. 1). Strong tranquilizers, such as Dalmane and Valium, are commonly overused and, because of the duration of their clinical actions, their effects may persist for longer periods of time in an older patient, resulting in lassitude, lack of thought and psychomotor coordination, and other side effects (see Julien 1988, pp. 58f.). Haldane and Mellaril are antipsychotic drugs used in nursing homes "to control behavior rather than treat a specific psychiatric illness" (Spiegel 1991, p. 20). Unless these and any other drugs are officially prescribed by a medical doctor to treat specific disorders, such usage is illegal, an indignity, and an immoral violation of patient rights. Clearly, for the protection of elder residents, legal intervention, punitive fines, and constant governmental supervision of treatment of residents in nursing homes are long overdue. One hesitates to continue to place responsibility for good and proper elder care solely under the aegis of governmental bodies. Of course, family members must become involved, but there are many elders who are absolutely alone, discarded and forgotten by family, and they need help and protection. Until we object to maltreatment, and until non-compliant nursing homes are brought under control, the mistreatment of elders will continue (see chapter 7).

ELDERS AND ALCOHOL

Some elders enjoy a glass of wine, a beer, or their evening cocktail. They find the drink relaxing, perhaps promoting sociability. Many see themselves as social drinkers; they know when to stop, and they are not particularly troubled if no liquor is available. They are in control. Others are not so fortunate: they are dependent on alcohol and must have their drinks. Some are heavy drinkers. Whether they admit it or not these elders are alcoholics. In the central nervous systems of both the social drinker and the alcoholic, alcohol exerts its influence as a depressant affecting performance skills—both mental and physical. We have all seen persons who reveal the effects of alcohol. Their speech becomes slightly slurred; their gait unsteady. The results of consuming alcohol can range from "mild social disinhibition to obnoxious buffoonery to sedation and sleep and finally to unconsciousness" (Forni 1978, p. 76).

How are we to distinguish between the social drinker and the alcoholic? Sometimes the differences are blurred because individuals react differently to alcohol. In other words, some elders "handle their booze" better than others. For our purpose, the distinctions are relatively unimportant, because if the elder is taking medications, any amount of alcohol may interact with the drugs and endanger the person's well-being. Many pharmacists include warnings on some prescriptions: "Check with MD before drinking alcohol." There is no suggestion in the warning about the amount of alcohol that is considered to be dangerous; the advice means "any alcohol."

The moral responsibility for the use, misuse, or abuse of drugs of any kind is primarily that of the elder for whom the medication is prescribed. The ethical responsibility for advising, instructing, cautioning, and warning the elder about the proper and improper use of medications and drugs must rest with the medical doctor and the pharmacist.

LEARNED DEPENDENCY

Just before his death, Norman Cousins (1990) wrote, "The worst thing about being 75 years old is being treated as a 75-year-old." He pointed out that earlier in his life, an airline hostess would simply hand him a blanket, but at seventy-five, they tucked him in. As an elder, he automatically received a discount at theaters. Cousins commented that "the greatest need of the elderly is to change the attitude of society toward aging." His observations are on target because society treats elders as enfeebled and in need of help; thus society educates its elders to act as if they are helpless.

To some degree and in some instances, society facilitates elder dependency. Martin Seligman (1975) demonstrated the reality of learned helplessness. When we treat the elderly as helpless human beings, it should come as no surprise that many do become helpless, and this learned behavior can hinder further growth and drain motivation. The stereotype of the helpless elder is both engendered and perpetuated. Even the Social Security system—a real life-saver for many elders—creates an image of older adults as depending on a fixed income. When these elders come for hospital treatment or nursing home care, the staff has already (stereotypically) catalogued them as dependent. Instead of creating a healthy mental response, these rehabilitative institutions facilitate illness. Elders begin to believe they actually are less than capable persons.

Recent studies demonstrate that hospitalized elders exhibit the highest rate of physical dependency. Of course this is to be expected, and one can assume that those receiving the most help are the very people in need of the most assistance. However, the hospital staff can compound dependency by their assumptions and mental attitudes regarding elderly patients. For example, when patients rate themselves on their abilities relating to eating, dressing, and toileting, their self evaluations are much higher than those of the caring staff. In a setting where patients learn that they will always be fed, bathed, clothed, and so forth regardless of their need, they conform to the anticipated pattern and an environment of dependency is created. Moreover, dependency engendered within the institution makes it harder for elders to cope and become independent once they are released from the hospital.

Part of the problem lies in the institutional notion of custodial care according to which elders must be provided full care because they are in the custody of the organization. The model of care may promote dependence since the interest of the staff is not in rehabilitation or encouraging independence but in care alone. The ideal institution approaches custodial care focused on the maintenance of the patient's independence wherever and whenever possible. In such a positive environment, elders are encouraged and rewarded by staff at all levels for their involvement in maintaining independent functioning.

Another contribution to learned dependency in hospitals and nursing homes is the emphasis on efficiency and the conservation of time and energy. Elders who feed themselves may require more time for eating than if they are fed. Those who wish to bathe and toilet themselves may not be as efficient or as thorough in self-care as they are when aided by staff persons. The institution is always fearful of accidents that can result in lawsuits, and elders who operate on their own can fall and injure themselves, which opens the facility to litigation. Operational ease and legal protection are important factors in institutional care, hence patient independence tends to become a secondary concern.

A similar pattern of developed elder dependency can appear when care is handled by the family. The statements "Don't let grandpa rake the leaves, he could hurt himself" or "Don't let grandma help with the dishes, she is too old to be doing such things" represent attitudes that rob elders of feelings of autonomy and capability. Because the elderly are "getting on in years" it is assumed that they automatically suffer from diminished ability. If an eighteen-year-old daughter breaks a dish, she has had an accident and ought to be more careful. If grandma were to break a dish, it is because she is too old and too unsteady to handle dishes.

The end result is that elders with physical ability are denied the opportunity to express that ability and are made dependent on the family.

Many family caregivers become overprotective of their resident elder. "Don't get up, I'll get it for you" tends to limit the elder's mobility and encourages passivity. Often well-meant overcare stifles the independence that is so necessary for physical well-being. For example, an elderly woman who complained of experiencing some difficulty in walking is taken by her son to a therapist. On arrival, the son opens the door, seats the elder and describes his mother's problem to the therapist—how she shuffles, how he feels it necessary to help her get about, how slow her gait has become, and so forth. The son ignores the fact that the problem is his mother's, and that while she may experience some difficulty in walking, there is nothing wrong with her ability to communicate. The therapist suggests an evaluation and the mother is interviewed alone. When the son returns, the therapist explains that there is really little that is physically wrong; the mother walks well and without assistance and only needs the opportunity and encouragement to move about on her own. The son is outraged. He knows something is wrong and he leaves with his mother who, the therapist notes, has resumed shuffling and is now leaning on his arm. In this instance of pseudo-physical dependency, the dependency is not that of the elder alone; the son has become dependent on this dependency. The elder provides the caregiver with a definite role, a sense of being needed and therefore important. Both the caregiver and elder are made emotionally dependent, and in the case of the elder, physical dependency exists as well.

Not every family is ready to examine the feelings that lie behind the encouragement of dependency in elders. The elderly relative joins the family of the son or daughter as "momma" or "grandma" or as "daddy" or "grandpa" and immediately becomes involved in a role reversal. The house is no longer the elder's home where the older person is responsible for the well-being of children; instead, the home is that of the child where feelings of responsibility for the well-being of one or more elders abounds. The intrusion of an elder into an established family setting can result in mixed feelings of frustration, anger, guilt, and anxiety. If the elder suffers from any impairment or illness, these feeling responses can be exacerbated. The family may pay little heed to what the elder may be experiencing within.

Counseling and therapy can be useful ways of resolving dependency problems. The open discussion of affect and emotions in a controlled setting provides opportunity for the exploration of ways to resolve problems. When elders have the will and the ability to help with household chores and when they can make some financial contribution toward household expenses, feelings of participation and self-maintenance are encouraged and the sense of dependency is reduced.

One can readily understand why some elders do not want to live with their children but prefer to be on their own. These elders may hobble around their own homes, doing what they can to maintain the environment, ignoring what seems unimportant (such as regular dusting and vacuuming), but in full awareness that they are still able to take care of themselves with limited assistance from the outside. One absolutely happy elder is pleased that she is able to live in her own home. Her children feel the place could stand some repair but they are willing to let the woman manage as she wishes. When newspapers and magazines pile up in one room, she simply hires a neighbor boy to put them out for the recycling team to pick up. She doesn't worry that the hallway or living room may be untidy with the stacks of old reading materials, she is not at home long enough to pay much attention to them. At the age of eighty-three she is too busy with outside activities to pay attention to such minor housekeeping details. She is independent and living her life as she wishes.

Another contributing factor to elder dependency lies in the Medicare and Medicaid systems that were designed to provide preventive medicine but actually offer only partial care inasmuch as they really focus on acute care. Health problems affecting elder functioning tend to be more often chronic than acute; they include, for example, decline of eyesight and hearing. Yet hearing aids and eyeglasses are not covered by Medicaid. Because the elder must be virtually housebound to qualify for aid, the assistance that would help to maintain independence and health is denied.

THE RIGHT TO KNOW

Professionals in health care face special ethical dilemmas. Patients' rights advocates emphasize the right of the patient to be informed as fully as possible about his or her disease or illness and be granted the freedom to make choices in treatment. Most doctors and hospitals have no problem with this principle, at least in general, but problems can arise when patients do not handle the information well. For example, Hugh R. K. Barber (1987) has noted:

When the patient is told that cancer is present, her immediate psychologic response is one of acute emotional turmoil, which may last from a few days to several days or weeks. Fortunately, as the patient assimilates the information and recovers from her shock, and perhaps disbelief about the diagnosis, she slowly begins to accept its reality. However, patients experience insomnia, anorexia, and difficulty in concentrating and work-ing following the diagnosis. There are differences in the way they react. The older patient is more inclined to develop depression, whereas the younger patient tends to express more anger and may be less cooperative as a result of this anger. She feels that society, her family, or her friends are at fault, or that she has been cursed for something that is beyond her control. The older patient immediately starts worrying about becoming a burden to others, the financial costs, and the loss of dignity. (p. 14)

One must assume that the responses described are not limited to female patients! Indeed, it would be a safe bet that most persons, regardless of age, react to the announcement that they have cancer with similar emotional and physical responses.

Inasmuch as some medical professionals may be troubled by these initial reactions, the medical problem assumes new ethical dimensions. "How to tell?" "When to tell?" and "How much to divulge?" are weighty questions and responsibilities that confront the physician (Kalra, Rosner, and Shapiro 1987, p. 20). Health experts must be sensitive teachers, realizing that patients may practice mental denial and do not always hear what they are told. Psychologists have pointed out that denial is a normal coping response that serves to distance a person from unpleasant and disturbing news. There is nothing destructive in denial other than that it becomes a source of annoyance to the medical profession, which would prefer patients to accept what they are told without expressing any of the well-known coping patterns, including depression, anger, and physical upset. What is needed is caring, patient reiteration of the information by the medical team.

Like most people, elders address such situations with a variety of responses. Some want to be informed about all possible side effects, all possible life trajectories, and every minute detail of their illness. In some instances, such information makes the patient a compliant and cooperative warrior against the disease; in other cases, the patient begins to worry about the future (which even the doctor cannot project) and interprets every muscle twitch as a prognosticator of the worst. A friend of mine gave her father a copy of the American Medical Association's excellent *Family Medical Guide,* which contains diagnostic charts. The result was disastrous. The man began to read the charts and, sure enough, he found that he had the symptoms of major ailments. A simple backache became evidence of a prolapsed disc, an itchy spot was dermatitis, a stiff shoulder was incipient bursitis, temporary hoarseness was a warning of tumor of the larynx, and so on. For some people a little information can become a dangerous diagnostic tool. Yet elders have the right to know, the right to participate in decisions concerning treatment and care, and the right not to be deceived or treated as children.

ETHICAL ISSUES IN HEALTH RESEARCH

Human fetal tissue research has become one of the smoldering issues confronting promising new investigations of diseases such as juvenile diabetes, leukemia, immune system disorders, as well as such illnesses as Parkinson's disease, Alzheimer's disease, and Huntington's disease, which directly affect elders. The Stanford University research on fetal tissue use reported that the benefits such studies "may bring cannot be guaranteed, but the opportunities to preserve life and alleviate suffering could be enormous" (Greenly 1989, p. 1093). Indeed, in Mexico City the condition of two Parkinson's victims improved markedly after surgeons grafted brain tissue from a miscarried fetus (Gorman 1988). Parkinson's disease results in the loss of the transmitter Dopamine in the brain and introduction of the fetal tissue prompted the production of the vital substance.

Of course, fetal tissues have been used during the past fifty years to develop self-sustaining cell lines used for diagnosis of disease and the production of human vaccines. "In fact, the discovery of the polio vaccine in the 1950s was based on cultures of human fetal kidney cells" (Cimons 1990). Recently the research has focused on "experimental surgery involving the transplanting of fetal cells—healthy cells that it is hoped will assume the functions of diseased or defective cells in the body" (Cimons 1990). "Three properties make human fetal tissue particularly useful in transplants: it grows rapidly, it is very adaptable, and when it is treated properly it evokes little or no immune response from the host" (Greenly 1989, p. 1093). Then what is the problem?

In April 1988, partially in response to protests from anti-abortion groups, the Ronald Reagan administration instituted a moratorium on federal funding of tissue research on aborted fetuses. Anti-abortionists argue that fetal tissue, obtained from what they consider to be an immoral procedure, is tainted; despite the potential for saving lives, in their view, it should not be used. The suggestion has also been made that knowledge of the use of fetal tissue for humanitarian purposes might encourage women who were as yet undecided to proceed with an abortion. Indeed, one Parkinson's victim declined his daughter's offer to get pregnant and then have an abortion to provide the needed fetal tissue for his treatment (Gorman 1988). A further complicating question might be whether a female who chooses abortion has any right to decide whether or not the aborted fetal tissue could be used for research.

Such arguments automatically lead to sanctity-of-life issues and to discussions as to whether or not the fetus is a person, i.e., a human being with moral and ethical rights. In an extreme view, it can be argued that the fetus is simply a part of the mother's body equivalent to a heart or kidney. It can be seen simply as tissue to be used as any other tissue would be used. A less extreme view evaluates the aborted fetus as a cadaver, subject to the Uniform Anatomical Gift Act of 1968, which means that it could be donated (Muyskens 1979, pp. 163f.). This view does not accept the fetus as a part of the moral community with moral responsibilities and choices, but does recognize the mother as a member with autonomy to make choices for herself and the fetal cadaver. Perhaps an ethical line might be drawn to not accept the production of fetuses simply for scientific experimentation, no matter how noble the cause or intention to benefit others.

What is ignored is the fact that the fetal tissues from the estimated 1.5 million abortions performed in the United States each year are almost all cremated or discarded. To destroy and waste tissue that could be used to help others can only be evaluated as a moral travesty. Of course some fetal cell research is carried on independently, but the potential health benefits will not be realized until fully funded studies are undertaken. At the time of writing, the struggle to remove the moratorium is still in initial stages. All the while, huge sums of money are being invested in the search for cures of the very diseases that fetal cell research gives promise of alleviating. Although one may object to the production of fetuses purely for research, inasmuch as abortion is considered legal, the use of aborted fetal material to help elders and others suffering from debilitating illnesses cannot be considered immoral or unethical. At this point, a utilitarian philosophical stance makes sense.

REFERENCES

The American Medical Association Home Medical Encyclopedia. 1989.
New York: Random House, 2 vols.

Ball, Avis Jane. 1986. *Caring for an Aging Parent: Have I Done All I Can?* Buffalo, N.Y.: Prometheus Books.

Barber, Hugh R. K. 1987. "Psychosocial Aspects of Chemotherapy," *Loss, Grief, and Care* 1, nos. 3/4 (Spring/Summer): 11–18.

Brady, Edward S. 1978. "Drugs and the Elderly," in Ronald C. Kayne, ed., *Drugs and the Elderly*. Los Angeles: University of Southern California Press, pp. 1–7.

Cassell, Christine, and Ruth B. Purtilo. 1981. *Ethical Dimensions in the Health Professions*. Philadelphia: W. B. Saunders Company.

Cimas, Marlene. 1990. "Waxman Seeks to Restore U.S. Funds for Human Cell Studies," *The Los Angeles Times,* August 8.

Cousins, Norman. 1990. "Don't Tuck Me In," *The Los Angeles Times,* December 3.

Dallek, Geraldine. 1990. "Health-Care System Will Continue to Die—Until More Feel the Pain," *The Los Angeles Times,* August 19.

Dean, Paul. 1990. "Doctor Accuses Another of Fraudulent Practices," *The Los Angeles Times,* July 31.

Forni, Peter J. 1978. "Alcohol and the Elderly," in Ronald C. Kayne, ed., *Drugs and the Elderly*. Los Angeles: University of Southern California Press, pp. 75–83.

Fox, Nancy. 1986. *You, Your Aging Parent, and the Nursing Home.* Buffalo, N.Y.: Prometheus Books.

Goldin, G., S. Perry, and R. Margolin. 1972. *Dependency and Its Implications for Rehabilitation.* Lexington, Mass.: Lexington Books.

Gollub, James. 1978. "Psychoactive Drug Misuse Among the Elderly: A Review of Prevention and Treatment Programs," in Ronald C. Kayne, ed., *Drugs and the Elderly*. Los Angeles: University of Southern California Press, pp. 84–102.

Gorman, Christine. 1988. "A Balancing Act of Life and Death," *Time,* February 1, p. 49.

Gorovitz, Samuel. 1982. *Doctor's Dilemmas—Moral Conflict and Medical Care.* New York: Macmillan Publishing Co.

Greenly, Henry T., et al. 1989. "Special Report: The Ethical Use of Human Fetal Tissue in Medicine," *The New England Journal of Medicine* 320, no. 16 (April): 1093–96.

Kapla, J., F. Rosner, and S. Shapiro. 1987. "Emotional Strain on Physicians Caring for Cancer Patients," *Loss, Grief and Care* 1, nos. 3/4 (Spring/Summer): 19–24.

Kemp, B., K. Brummel-Smith, and J. Ramsdell. 1990. *Geriatric Rehabilitation.* Boston: College-Hill Press.

Kugler, Hans J. 1977. *Slowing Down the Aging Process.* New York: Jove/
    Harcourt Brace Jovanovich.
Insight. 1988a. "The Specter of Rationing," August 8, p. 12.
Insight. 1988b. "Medicine Minus a Cost Tourniquet," August 8, pp. 8–14.
Johnson, Ted, and Marla Cone. 1990. "EPA Cites Marines for Waste
    Handling," *The Los Angeles Times,* Orange County edition, August 9.
Julien, Robert M. 1988. *A Primer of Drug Action,* 5th ed. New York:
    W. H. Freeman and Company.
Lofholm, Paul. 1978. "Self-Medication by the Elderly," in Ronald C. Kayne,
    ed., *Drugs and the Elderly.* Los Angeles: University of Southern Cali-
    fornia Press, pp. 8–28.
Melmon, Kenneth L., and Howard F. Morelli. 1972. *Clinical Pharmacology.*
    New York: Macmillan Publishing Co.
Menzel, Paul T. 1983. *Medical Costs, Moral Choices.* New Haven, Conn.:
    Yale University Press.
Moody, H. R. 1985. "A Scenario for the Future? Rationing Medical
    Resources on the Grounds of Age," *Generations* 10, pp. 43f.
Muyskens, James L. 1979. "Cadaver Organs for Transplantation," *Human
    Life Controversies and Concerns.* New York: The H. W. Company.
Pearlman, R. A. 1985. "The Use of Quality of Life Considerations in Med-
    ical Decision Making," *Journal of the American Gerontological Society*
    33, pp. 342–51.
Quinn, W., and G. Hughston. 1984. *Independent Aging: Family and Social
    Systems Perspectives.* Rockville, Md.: Aspen Publications.
Rashkis, H. 1981. *Caring for Aging Parents.* Philadelphia: Stickley Co.
Roan, Shari. 1990. "Researchers Try to Raise Quality of Extended Life,"
    The Los Angeles Times, March 3.
Seligman, M. 1975. *Helplessness: On Depression, Development, and Death.*
    New York: W. H. Freeman & Company.
Skinner, B. F. 1972. "Compassion and Ethics in the Care of the Retardate,"
    Cumulative Record: A Selection of Papers, 3d ed. New York: Meredith
    Corporation, pp. 283–91.
Spiegel, Claire. 1991. "Restraints, Drugging, Rife in Nursing Homes," *The
    Los Angeles Times,* March 25.
van Praag, H. M. 1978. *Psychotropic Drugs.* New York: Brunner/Mazel,
    Inc.
Wade, B. L. Sawyer, and J. Bell. 1983. *Dependency with Dignity.* London:
    Bedford Square Press.
Walsh, Mary Williams. 1990. "Health System in Canada Cuts Costs and
    Care," *The Los Angeles Times,* April 9.

Wielawski, Irene. 1990. "Cuts in Funding Force Clinics to Turn Away People in Need," *The Los Angeles Times,* September 10.

———. 1991. "Significant Deterioration in Health of U.S. Children Found," *The Los Angeles Times,* March 12.

Winslow, Gerald R. 1982. *Triage and Justice.* Los Angeles: University of California Press.

Yarbough, Mark. 1988. "Continued Treatment of the Fatally Ill for the Benefit of Others," *Journal of the American Gerontological Society* 36.

Zarit, Stephen H., Nancy K. Orr, and Judy M. Zarit. 1985. *The Hidden Victims of Alzheimer's Disease: Families Under Stress.* New York: New York University Press.

15

Dementing Illness—
When the Mind Begins to Go

"The dementias are the most devastating and dreaded disorders of later life."

—Zarit, Orr, and Zarit, *The Hidden Victims of Alzheimer's Disease: Families Under Stress,* p. 1

"I can't find my keys. I must be getting old!" The common folklore that forgetfulness is a necessary aspect of aging is nonsense. Many elders have memories that are as keen and retentive as younger persons. Our memory patterns differ from person to person. One of my university professors had a photographic memory. He could drive me to distraction by quoting almost word for word sections out of books he had read years earlier. He made me feel that he was using parts of his brain that I had not discovered in mine. A colleague used to be able to identify by name every student in his class of over one hundred after they had indicated their names during the first session. It took me the best part of a semester to know the names of some thirty students in my classes. Occasionally someone will undertake to retain names through a process of association. At a party, one young man was introduced to a woman whose last name was "Horn." He associated her in his mind with the brass section of an orchestra. On their next meeting he struggled in his mind through "Miss Cornet," "Miss Bugle," and "Miss Trumpet" before giving up! In other words, each of us has different memory patterns. Growing old is not concomitant with loss of memory.

On the other hand, there are dementing illnesses associated with aging in which loss of memory may be involved. These illnesses can place tremendous burdens on caregivers, for when a frail elder is cognitively impaired the burden of care is compounded. Presently, it is estimated that up to four million people suffer from some form of dementia. As the population ages, the number of those with dementing illnesses will increase and more people will be cast into the role of caregivers.

Dementia is not a disease. The term refers to a group of symptoms that characterize a steady loss of mental powers in otherwise alert individuals. Two major conditions are responsible for the symptoms of confusion, memory loss, disorientation, and so forth. The first is delirium, which is often referred to as "acute brain syndrome" or "reversible brain syndrome," and which makes the person less alert or seemingly drowsy. This condition can be caused by illnesses such as pneumonia or kidney infection or by reactions to medications or by malnutrition. In many cases delirium can be successfully treated (Mace and Rabins 1981).

The second condition related to dementia causes intellectual impairment in a person who is clearly awake. Mental impairment progresses from forgetfulness to total disability. The most common disorders that cause irreversible dementia include Alzheimer's Disease, multi-infarct dementia, and Pick's Disease. Others, to name just a few, are Parkinson's Disease,* Huntington's Disease,† and Jakob-Creutzfeldt Disease.‡ One other form of dementia may result from depression and is, therefore, reversible by treatment. We will briefly consider only Alzheimer's Disease, multi-infarct dementia, and Pick's Disease.

The most common form of dementia is produced by Alzheimer's Disease (hereafter referred to as AD). Because AD cannot be truly confirmed until an autopsy is performed, the usual diagnosis is senile dementia of the Alzheimer's type, abbreviated as SDAT (Miner et al. 1989). AD is

---

*Parkinson's Disease is a brain disorder causing muscle tremors (trembling), stiffness, weakness, fatigue, and in some cases memory loss and dementia. It appears to result from a lack of dopomine (a nerve transmitter in the brain) due to degeneration of the nerve cell clusters known as the basal ganglia. It is treated with levodopa (L-Dopa).

†Huntington's Disease is also caused by degeneration of the basal ganglia, which results in *chorea* (rapid, jerky, involuntary grimaces and twitches) affecting the face and arms, and dementia. There is no known cure for the disease, but some lessening of chorea may result from use of the drug chlorpromazine. The greatest help seems to result from good, loving, nursing care.

‡Jakob-Creutzfeldt Disease is a relatively rare form of late-life dementia that appears to be caused by a viral agent. The disease is progressive and there is no cure.

marked by specific structural changes in the brain including senile plaques (degenerated cell structures), neurofibrillary tangles (masses of tangled fibers that partially displace normal cell structures), brain atrophy in the frontal and temporal lobes, and overall loss of neurons (or brain cells). In the examination of autopsied brains of normal elders, these conditions are rarely found; they are abundant in the brains of dementia patients.

What are the symptoms of AD? They include gradual declines in memory, learning ability, attention span, judgment, time and space orientation, accessing words and communicating them, and changes in personality (Aronson 1988). Because the symptoms may be vague at first, the victim may be able to make compensations and disguise the ailment. As the disease progresses the normal aspects of memory progressively fail. Normal patterns break down and those with AD may need to be reminded to brush their teeth or wash their hands. Speech impairment such as dysphasia—the inability to arrange words in the proper sequence—becomes apparent. Sometimes movement coordination is affected (dyspraxia). There are difficulties in reading and writing and in the ability to carry on a normal conversation. Often victims will wander and become lost in familiar territory: for example, they may be unable to find the bathroom, their bedroom, or the front door to exit in an emergency. If they stray outside of the home, they could become completely disoriented.

By the time the final stages of AD are reached tremendous damage has been done to the brain tissue: almost all mental functions are disrupted or disturbed and most victims require constant supervision. They cannot perform most daily activities and there is fecal and urinary incontinence. Conversations are impossible, and often close relatives and spouses are not recognized. Ultimately victims need assistance with all aspects of daily living. Some become bedridden. Ultimately, they die.

Multi-infarct dementia, the second most common cause of dementia, results from repeated strokes caused by small occlusions or artery blockages within the cortical and subcortical parts of the brain; the blockages destroy small areas within these regions of the brain. Memory, coordination, and speech are usually affected, but the symptoms differ according to the location of the brain strokes and the size of the blocked artery. Although the symptoms mimic those of AD, multi-infarct dementias progress in a step-like way as opposed to the gradual decline in AD. The causes are unknown but risk factors involved are similar to those associated with heart disease and strokes including high blood pressure, high cholesterol diet, overweight, smoking, and lack of exercise (Zarit et al. 1985). While there is no way to reverse the disease, it is clear that elders can take the health precautions that are known to negate strokes, high blood pressure, and so forth.

The onset of Pick's Disease is rapid and the progression is much faster than AD or multi-infarct dementia. Personality changes are more in evidence in the beginning stages and memory loss and spatial impairment soon follow. There is no cure for this disease, which affects the temporal or frontal lobes of the brain.

Many elders are deeply troubled by the onset of these diseases. They know something is wrong, that something is happening to them. They feel confused, helpless, isolated, and perhaps angry with themselves for their failure to operate as usual. Some skillfully conceal the fact that something is wrong. They make excuses that sound reasonable. They divert attention from their failures. They write notes reminding themselves of things to be done. They avoid social situations where their limitations might become obvious. Informed elders who know something about dementia may seek to discover all they can about the ailment by using library facilities and questioning professionals. They desire to clear the confusion and to find a label for what is troubling them.

When Janet Adkins of Portland, Oregon, discovered that she had Alzheimer's Disease, she took her own life while still in the early stages of the disease. Mrs. Adkins is remembered as a healthy activist fifty-seven-year-old, an educator who prized her physical and mental abilities. She knew about AD and had no intention of letting the disease run its full course. She had read about the so-called suicide machine invented by Dr. Jack Kevorkian, and while she was still able to make decisions and after considerable consultation with Kevorkian and her family physician, as well as a psychiatrist, she utilized the machine to terminate her life. Her suicide was condemned by those who felt that she could have waited longer before taking her life since she could have had many good years left. Others applauded Mrs. Adkins's decision as coinciding with their own feelings of not wanting to lose the mental dimensions that give savor to life, and of not wishing to become a living burden that others would have to carry.

There can be no question that dementia places burdens on families and caregivers. Some victims regress to childlike behavior, while others throw tantrums that can be frightening, particularly if the person is physically strong. Still others are simply bewildered by everything that goes on around them. As the disease moves into its mature phases, victims cannot be left alone. They can be dangerous to themselves and others. For example, one AD victim would turn on the gas jets in the stove whenever possible, endangering the lives of the family. Another would slip away and head for refuse bins behind supermarkets to find damaged fruit which the person then handed out to children in the street. The need for constant vigilance can wear down the best of caregivers.

What resources are available? In the early stages, family members are usually able to cope with dementia. The elder requires only minimal supervision and can participate in limited ways in family life. As the need for supervision increases, caregivers can be employed to look after the patient when the family is not home. But because caregivers are often hired on a hit-or-miss basis, inadequately prepared or poorly trained individuals may cause more problems than they solve. Ultimately, the elder may have to be institutionalized.

There can be little question that the most satisfying and most healthful environment for the ailing elder is the home. Familiarity of surroundings, sounds, food, and associations does seem, in some cases, to delay the progress of the dementia. But the problems for caregivers can become overwhelming. Personal items of family members may be taken and misplaced. The elder may no longer recognize his or her spouse. One female AD victim screamed in terror when her husband entered her room; she no longer knew who he was. A male AD sufferer threw everything he could lay his hands on at his son who he thought was an intruder in the home.

Although some claim that the dementia victim seems to decline faster in institutional settings, others find that the elder adapts rapidly and easily. One elder, whose husband no longer recognized her, discovered that he had found a "girlfriend" in the institution where he had been placed. At first she was shocked and troubled seeing him walking hand-in-hand with the female resident, but then she had to admit to herself: "The man I married is dead. This is only a physical shell of the person. If he finds some sort of happiness with his 'girlfriend'—a happiness which he cannot have with me, I can only wish him well."

Group sessions for caregivers of dementia victims can provide help in developing coping skills. First caregivers find that they are not alone and that others face similar situations in their efforts to give love and support to ailing family members. Guilt feelings associated with abandoning the elder to institutional care may be assuaged through sharing. Tensions are lessened as caregiver after caregiver relates the most ridiculous situations that occur in their household or with their patient. Ways of handling problem situations are shared. Advice is given and literature and helpful films are discussed. Supportive friendships develop.

The ethical issues arise out of family loyalty. What should family members do when dementia strikes an elder? How long should the family bear the responsibility for care that disrupts the normal lives of those in the household and adds pressure to their already stressful existence? Is it ethical to place elders who suffer from one of the many forms of dementia in an institution?

Of course there can be no single answer to these questions. The ethical response will vary according to the situation. Some families (relatives or spouses) never question that they have a personal responsibility for the care of a family member, no matter how disrupting the ailment may be to their familial existence. For others, who feel equally responsible but who also recognize their own limitations, the most compassionate and ethical act is to place the elder where the best care is available—care that surpasses that available in a home setting. Familial loyalty calls for regular visits to institutionalized elders, even when the visitors are no longer recognized or appreciated. For younger members of the family, the notion of their parents experiencing being orphaned while the grandparents are still alive but dead to familial relationships makes no sense. To some family members it is a waste of time to visit someone who can't recognize them and who doesn't care whether or not they are there. Others may empathize with their parents' anguish at losing parental elders, but feel that their own lives take precedent over concern for elders who are mentally dead.

The suicidal end chosen by Janet Adkins has triggered responses from some who would also choose death rather than life as an AD victim. But Kevorkian's machine has been placed legally off limits, and therefore that particular choice does not exist. Those whose families have a history of dementia look to science to find a way to halt these devastating diseases of the mind and ultimately to cure them once they have started. Certainly continuing and extensive governmental, medical, and pharmaceutical support of research is called for as a humane and ethical response to a dire disease. Meanwhile other ethical considerations include:

- careful and accurate diagnosis so that the dementia will be correctly recognized and properly treated;

- humane care that guarantees comfort and security for victims of these dread diseases;

- compassionate response to and support of family members and of those responsible for ailing elders.

REFERENCES

Aronson, Miriam K. 1987. *Understanding Alzheimer's Disease.* New York: Macmillan Publishing Co.

Breslau, Lawrence D., and Marie R. Haug, eds. 1983. *Depression and Aging.* New York: Springer Publishing Company.

Brown, Dorothy S. 1984. *Handle With Care: A Question of Alzheimer's.* Buffalo, N.Y.: Prometheus Books.

Carstensen, Laura L., and Barry A. Edelstein, eds. 1987. *Handbook of Clinical Gerontology.* New York: Pergamon Press.

Dippel, Raye Lynne, and J. Thomas Hutton, eds. 1991. *Caring for the Alzheimer Patient: A Practical Guide,* 2d ed. Buffalo, N.Y.: Prometheus Books.

Mace, N. L., and P. V. Rabins. 1981. *The 36-Hour Day.* Baltimore: The Johns Hopkins University Press.

Miner, J. D., et al. 1989. *Caring for Alzheimer's Patients.* New York: Plenum Press.

Zarit, Steven H. 1980. *Aging and Mental Disorders.* New York: The Free Press.

Zarit, S. H., N. K. Orr, and J. M. Zarit. 1985. *The Hidden Victims of Alzheimer's Disease: Families Under Stress.* New York: New York University Press.

16

Geroethics and Elder Sex

"Old men shave in the morning; young men shave in the evening."

—Folkloric saying

"Old people love less—and mean it more. Old people have intercourse less often—after a couple of coronaries, or when taking diuretics—but they feel deeply, nevertheless."

—Martin Grotjahn, in *Death: Current Perspectives,* p. 256

The folkloric saying quoted above reflects Puritanism and Victorian notions concerning sex that were prevalent at the beginning of this century, when elders were very young. No careful research into sex and aging had been done. Current attitudes toward elder sex, reflected in everything from jokes, stories about impotence, and religious beliefs served to encourage the notion that sexual impulses and relationships died or ceased or, perhaps, should have died or ceased, with aging. In those instances where elders continued to be sexually active, the behavior was either kept secret or treated with distance as socially abhorrent, giving rise to epithets like "dirty old man" and "shameless old woman." Perhaps the forty-seven-year life expectancy at the turn of the century suggested that sexual feelings died about the same age, thus any one who lived beyond that age and continued to express interest in sex was not normal. Martin Grotjahn's statement, echoed by many elders, reflects a reality, namely, that when today's life expectancy is in the mid-seventies, sexual feelings and responses do not cease with age. Unfortunately, despite courses in sex education, outmoded sexual attitudes still abound among those who should know better.

The danger is that some elders may buy into the negative stereotypes. If they believe there is something wrong with having sexual desires and longings, they may feel compelled to sublimate their feelings and deny what is now acknowledged as "normal." They may begin to feel that they are "too old" and thereby become subject to the sexual stereotypes of agism.

What lies behind the negativity toward elder sex? Perhaps prudish and up-tight attitudes toward sex in general may be traced to the ways in which some sects and denominations interpret the Bible or selected parts of the Bible. According to this thinking, sexual intercourse is for procreation only, the enjoyment is secondary. To engage in sex for pleasure alone is to violate religious precepts.

Perhaps our culture has absorbed some selected religious notions suggesting that sex is not quite clean (see "The Madonna-Whore" in Larue 1983, p. 71f). Sex, according to some biblical teachings, was something done in the night that left the couple unclean (see Lev. 15:16–18). Influenced by this kind of religious instruction, there are those who accept marital sex as a rather messy obligation. This was made clear to me when a student assistant told me that she had put off her marriage for the third time. When I asked why, she sighed and explained that it was because of sex. In subsequent conversations, it became clear that she had absolutely no understanding of sexual intercourse as an act or expression of love, nor was she informed about her own body or of the body of her fiance. Her very strict, religious mother had told her over and over again that sex was dirty and was a woman's duty to her husband. I was not surprised to find that this student was an only child! Then I learned that her grandmother had told both the mother and the student exactly the same thing, and sure enough, she, too, had only one child. I suggested to the young woman that she read some of the current books on sex, and in my mind I wished her a happy, successful, and sexually fulfilling marriage. I received one letter from her a year after the wedding. The young couple were living in another state and she was pregnant. I could not help wondering if this was to be the only child and whether through the modern literature about love, marriage, and sex she found in the books, plus her own natural feelings and responses, she would be able to overcome the educational contamination provided by her mother and grandmother. People act out what they believe about themselves. If they think negatively about sex and are convinced that sex has no place in the lives of elders, they will judge the sex lives of others according to these standards. There can be little doubt that there are others whose religious notions and biblical interpretations negatively affect the potential for full and free enjoyment of human sexuality. But other interpretations of biblical materials are possible.

At least one section of the Bible, the "Song of Songs," reflects joyous anticipation of and delight in human love-making. It is true that at one time some religious savants argued that the writings reflected the love of God for his people in Israel, or of Christ for his church, but modern scholarship has pretty well dispelled the validity of these interpretations. The poems may have originated in ancient fertility cult rituals, in which case they represent the dialogue between the male and female deities. Or they may have been part of ancient wedding rites (Larue 1983, chap. 29). In any case, it is clear that the amorous language is the language of human love.

As we have noted, elder sexuality is not disparaged in the Bible. The legends about Abraham and Sarah, and the fiction about prediluvian characters indicates that they produced children when they were in their hundreds (Gen. 5)!

The tendency to discount elder sex may be related to what Butler and Lewis (1976) called "aesthetic narrowness" in their discussion of the pressures placed on aging women (p. 6). As I will note later in the brief commentary on the film *Harold and Maude,* there are those who cannot see beauty in aged women (or in aged men) and the very thought of sex with someone who lacks the fresh vitality of youth becomes repulsive. As this form of "aesthetic narrowness" permeates and biases public thinking, elder sex becomes socially unacceptable and even unthinkable. Some years ago, a poster relating to the aged pictured an elderly man and woman engaged in an amorous kiss. Many found it "disgusting" or "repulsive." Why? Because of "aesthetic narrowness"?

Many sexually active young men and women in my university classes have difficulty imagining their parents making love—an activity that one student referred to as "humping." Indeed, that negation is so common that Doris B. Hammond titled her book *My Parents Never Had Sex* (1987)! Nor are these same youth able to imagine their parents experimenting with premarital sex. But there are others who entertain a different perspective. One young woman announced, "My mother and my granny are both very sexy ladies. They are my role models and when I am in my late sixties I plan to be just as sexy and just as sexually active as they are!" Great!

Some years ago, after class, I joined a few of the talented and creative young people from The Center for Art and Design in Pasadena for a late afternoon snack at a nearby bistro. In an adjoining booth, a group of men in business suits were into serious beer drinking conversation. They had loosened their ties, one had shed his jacket, and their voices were loud enough for us to listen in on a dialogue about sex and aging. One commented, "Well I am going to be forty years old next year and you know what that means—sex is going to be on the decline from then on." Another introduced the subject of menopause and announced that his wife was nearing the magical age of forty when, he informed his colleagues, all female sexual impulses die and, in his words, "Sex is dead." The conversation became important for the students. We had discussed aging and sex in class. They had become acquainted with the research of Masters and Johnson, Kinsey, Helen Singer Kaplan, and other sex researchers. They had learned that "The potential for erotic pleasure seems to begin with birth and does not need to end until death" (Kaplan 1974, p. 104). First, they smiled as they joked about the surprises awaiting the misinformed men in the next booth. Next, they talked about sex stereotypes applied to elders. Then they grasped the importance of their role as those who would be involved in advertising, which is a form of public education, and the importance of changing stereotypes that would one day impact on their own aging.

THE NURSING HOME SETTING

The belief that sex dies with the menopause or at some fixed age has been reenforced by the notion that sex *ought* to end for elders. An official of a retirement home run by a Christian denomination told me of an elderly couple who were interested in becoming residents. When they were shown accommodations with twin beds, the woman immediately said, "We have been sleeping together for forty years and we have no intention of sleeping in separate beds now. We want one bed, queen-sized." The middle-aged woman who was showing them the room sniffed and said, "I would have thought you two would be past all that nonsense by now."

Another supervisor told me of a problem that emerged after the hiring of a nineteen-year-old man who was slightly retarded to help with some of the heavier work in the residence. He was a big, attractive fellow with a kind and helpful attitude toward the residents. Then complaints filtered into the administrator's office. Some of the elderly women were startled when they found him standing in a linen closet, or walking in the halls at unusual times. One stated that she saw him trying to open the door of the room of one of the resident women but he left ("ran off" she said) when he saw her. Obviously, the management had to respond—the young man was fired.

"Then," said the manager, "complaints really came in." It seems the young man was, in the manager's words, "servicing" some of the elderly women, and they resented his dismissal. Because this residency was run by a church organization, the director was not free to sanction such behavior. "Therefore," the manager said, "the ladies went back to masturbation."

Perhaps the lack of awareness of and concern for the sexual needs of patients in nursing homes occurs "because nursing homes are geared more to needs and desires of families and smooth institutional operation than desires of patients . . . and the fact that most nursing home patients are usually without spouse and somewhat or totally immobile, makes any kind of socialization (let alone sexual gratification) somewhat of a challenge" (Steffl, pp. 147f). Cooper (1981) notes that because direct care staff are "generally untrained in human growth and development and often without sufficient supervisory guidance," they are "prone to insensitive responses to the common human needs of patients" (p. 506f). He comments further that "little serious attention is paid to sexuality by physicians, nurses, aides, or families, which reinforces repression and conflict in the elderly patient (p. 507).

In many nursing homes patient privacy is all but ignored. Staff members enter rooms without knocking (or knock and open the door in almost the same gesture). For two residents to share a bed and hold and caress each other in comfort requires the security of privacy. Few facilities provide intimacy rooms which elders can reserve to be alone with their visitors and feel secure enough in their privacy to kiss, hug, fondle, and perhaps engage in intercourse. Of course, there might be some embarrassment in making the reservation. Residents would know or perhaps guess what might be happening within the room. Obviously, the best solution is for residents to have their own private rooms where they can entertain guests and where staff members and other residents cannot enter without invitation, except perhaps in an emergency.

Sexual urges and feelings are alive in nursing home settings. One of my students, a very attractive young woman, was visiting a relative in a nursing home. As she walked down the corridor, an elderly man in a wheelchair spoke to her. She could not understand what he said, so she leaned down and put her ear closer to his mouth. At that moment he reached up and pulled her v-necked sweater down so he could peer in at her breasts. She was shocked and startled, but she was also mature in understanding. She realized that in his own way, this rather forward elder was making the statement that he was still a sexual human being. As she walked away she heard him giggle. In many ways institutional life is a microcosm of the broader society in which it is placed. As Cooper notes:

> Sexuality in an institution covers the same wide range of cognition, affect, and behavior as it does in the communities in which patients were reared and from which they entered the nursing home. It includes sexual fantasies, thoughts, dreams, jokes, discussions, hand-holding, kissing, touching, masturbation, exhibitionism, voyeurism, homosexuality, and intercourse. (1981, p. 507)

When elders enter an institution they do not automatically lose their sexual feelings. There is no reason from them to give up their rights to freedom of sexual expression. Of course, institutions must differentiate between accepted normal sexual drives that can be accommodated or ignored and problem behavior requiring intervention. Crude language as well as provocative and intrusive behavior can be upsetting to residents and staff. Dulcy B. Miller suggested that long-term care facilities, in keeping with federal regulations concerning patients' rights, need "to develop policies regarding sexual practices of inpatients including homosexual and heterosexual activity between brain-intact and brain-damaged residents" (p. 164). She presents five possible courses of action. One would be a hands-off approach: "sex is a private matter to be determined by each resident for himself irrespective of his intellectual capacity, with no interference from administration" (ibid.). The second, a laissez-faire approach, would encourage residents to "do their own thing," thereby, depending on the ethical and social stance of the management, providing "passive encouragement or discouragement to sexual activities of inpatients" (ibid.). A third suggestion was that the institution may act *in loco infantis,* with the wishes of the residents' children determining acceptable sexual behavior. On the other hand, in the fourth alternative, "The long-term care agency may actively encourage sexual fulfillment by patients as an important means of communication—as an activity to humanize the institution." If the goal for long-term care patients is a full, rich life, it follows that sex among patients should be sought actively" (ibid.). The final alternative offers the most restrictive option: "The nursing home may impose restraints on the sexual practices of residents in the belief that sex for the aged is unnatural and what is not natural is not good. Perhaps only certain publicly visible sex acts should be prohibited. Perhaps only senile patients should be protected from sexual involvement" (ibid.). Which is the ethical choice?

Of course, there must be concern for the sexuality of impaired individuals who have lost impulse control and who could pose dangers to others. But for those elders who are emotionally and physically and psychologically intact, the central ethical issue relating to elder sex in institutional settings has to do with institutional rights versus elder rights. Elders, like anyone else, have the constitutional right to privacy. The institution also has rights, and its policies should be made clear before the elder becomes a resident. If the institutional intent is to limit or forbid elder expressions of sexual feelings, these restrictions should be clearly and explicitly spelled out before the elder is admitted. On the other hand, if elder rights to the expression of sexual feelings are permissible, then privacy and the provision of places for privacy are imperative. What is often forgotten is that for the resident elder the nursing home becomes "home" and unless the freedom to express oneself sexually, in the kind of privacy one would enjoy in one's own home, is respected and available, the nursing home becomes something less than a "home" and functions as a confining and restricting institution.

Clearly, there is need among professionals as well as among the general public for a great deal of education concerning elder sex before attitudes are likely to change. According to Eric Pfeiffer:

> Attitudinally, physicians need to understand that aging patients retain their right to sexual expression, if need be in altered form and in altered settings, and that they also retain their right to ask for and receive professional counsel when they encounter difficulties in their legitimate pursuits for satisfying sexual expression. It is quite clear that many physicians and other health care personnel share with the rest of society a distinct taboo regarding sexual expression on the part of aging individuals. (1978, p. 27)

Staff members must be trained so that there will be none of the snickering and wise-cracking that Carlfred Broderick encountered while discussing a book dealing with this topic during a meeting with social workers, psychiatrists, and psychologists in a Veterans Administration hospital. He found that for these "people helpers" "the concept of sex after sixty was a joke" (1978, p. 7).

Some nursing home residents have commented on the need to be "sneaky" about sexual feelings, particularly if their feelings are for a partner of the same sex. Like many in our present society, some caregivers are uneasy and uncomfortable with, or are hostile to, homosexuality. Women touching or caressing or sleeping with women, or men touching and caressing and sleeping with men are considered to be abnormal. In the privacy of their own homes, lesbian and homosexual elders can live together comfortably; in residential settings, however, their feelings and love for one another can be deemed unacceptable. Derogatory labels ("old faggot," "old queen," "old dyke") make homosexuals and lesbians feel like outcasts, isolated from the larger residential family. Once again, privacy and the right to be one's own sexual self are important ethical dimensions in residential settings as well as in society at large.

THE OTHER 95 PERCENT

Most elders are not in institutions. About 95 percent live on their own, or with friends or family. It is not surprising to find that opposition to elder sex is not limited to institutions. Quite often "adult children . . . view their aged parents' normal urges for intimacy and romance as a threat of social disgrace and/or onset of second childhood" (Sviland, p. 98). When widowed parents begin to date they often become objects of concern for their adult children, who frown on intimacy and sometimes suggest that a sexual involvement is tantamount to infidelity to a dead spouse. The children may worry that should a marriage take place, the new partner may seek to control the widowed person's property. The fact is that in many, if not most, elder marriages, prenuptial contracts spell out inheritance rights.

Where no partners are available, the elder does what sexually motivated persons have done through the ages—he or she masturbates. Depending on religious training and inherited social mores, the act may or may not produce feelings of guilt. Adult children often find it difficult to imagine that their parents masturbate. One adult child was "shocked and horrified" when the single parent was "caught" masturbating. Although (pointing to the head) the adult child could accept the fact that the sexual organs remain sensitive and that sexual feelings might still be alive, on the other hand (pointing to the stomach) the gut reaction was disturbing. An interesting question was raised by this adult child: Why couldn't the elder get involved in some activities that would release tensions in a socially acceptable way rather than indulging in what the adult child called "self-abuse"? The notion of sublimation is not new. It has been part of Roman

Catholic teaching for celibate clergy for centuries, but it doesn't have to be the pattern adopted by elders. One might raise a question as to whether the adult child ever masturbated and whether his masturbation was also "self-abuse." If he did masturbate and accepted his own actions as "normal," then the distaste expressed at his parent's masturbating was nothing more than another example of "agism."

On every side we are confronted with a reality that informs, contrary to folklore, that sexual feelings, sexual desires, and the ability to respond sexually do not disappear with age. When a friend who was in his middle eighties married a woman in her late fifties, there were those who wondered about their sexual relations. The woman had been married and divorced and during the time of her single status had enjoyed numerous lovers. When one of her friends introduced the question of sex, she claimed that the eighty-year-old was "like a young stallion." Another friend, an expert in the study of sex, commented that the old stallion responded to a new filly, and that such responses were not uncommon among elders, even those who had been widowed and single for many years.

How do we deal with the confusion in the minds of some concerning aging and sex? How do we educate those who are ignorant of what is now known about human sexuality? First, it is important to emphasize that we are sexual beings by the very nature of our bodies whether or not our inclinations are directed toward members of the same sex or the opposite sex. Clifford and Joyce Penner (1981), are trained sex therapists who, as Christians, are confidant that "theology and biblical truths are not in conflict with current psychological understanding; rather the latter function as endorsements, confirmations, and amplifications of the scriptural teaching" (p. 22). While they would not endorse homosexuality, they recognize our sexual nature and inclinations: "We are sexual beings by creation," basing their argument on Genesis 1:27, where it is noted that human creation involved both "male and female" (p. 35).

Of course sexual expressions and relationships are not limited to intercourse. Touching, hand-holding, kissing, hugging, caressing, eye contact, intimate and warm conversations, and sharing food can all be sexual expressions between members of the same or opposite sex. Most people have little problem with elders walking arm-in-arm or holding hands. Some find elders kissing one another in anything other than a casual peck on the cheek or the lips to be upsetting. Other observers are embarrassed when elders flirt with one another. Two elders in a rather secluded part of a public park were, in the words of some members of their age-group, "carrying on in a disgusting manner" when they were involved in rather passionate kissing and fondling. Had they been young, the "carrying on" would have been dismissed as the passion of youth. We are not schooled to accept romantic love or passion between elders.

Movie and television screens portray young couples attempting to devour one another with amorous kisses. These same screens never show passionate elders engaged in the same activity. In the movie, *Harold and Maude* in which teenaged Harold fell in love with and had intercourse with the eighty-year-old Maude, the relationship was denigrated by Harold's mother and the priest who described his image of Maude's body in terms of disgust. The movie *On Golden Pond* depicted the relationship between Henry Fonda and Katharine Hepburn in an "appropriate" way. The feelings expressed were warm and caring but avoided any hint of intimacy or display of passion between the two elders. Why? Perhaps film makers, like many of us, believe that elders are supposed to have burned out the fires of passions and only youth can be sexually vigorous. Perhaps elders are supposed to be "dignified" and models of deportment suggesting that life has moved beyond the impulsive and passionate into reflective and controlled behavior.

It is true that for some elders sexual intimacy is not very important. For example, one couple had intimacy problems because the woman had never really liked sex. She had no knowledge of procreation until she was in her mid-twenties, despite a college education and a brief term served with the military. She married and had children, but although she had experienced and enjoyed orgasm, she had always felt that she had submitted to sex. Her husband, whom she still loved, was frustrated and confused. He was still sexually attracted to his wife and at sixty-four felt sexually vigorous. Their attitudes toward intimacy differed. She liked to be held and cuddled in bed, but if his hands began to "wander" or if she felt his erect penis pressing against her, she became uncomfortable and pushed him away. The point is that not every elder desires intercourse.

Separate bedrooms do not necessarily mean no sexual intimacy. As one woman explained: "He snores so loudly that he keeps me awake. Besides, it is kind of adventuresome to sneak down the hall into his bedroom to make love."

There are instances when a partner may be impotent, but unless the impotency is caused by physical reasons or perhaps by medically prescribed drugs, the triggering factors may be fatigue or mental reservations. Broderick has noted that retirement can induce feelings of loss of masculine status that can lead to impotence (1978, p. 5). For example, one male elder retired at age sixty-five after a serious heart bypass operation. Because he had made some poor investments, his retirement income was drastically reduced and he was terribly upset with himself. He had been widowed for twenty years and during that period was, in his words, "quite a ladies' man." He was popular and, despite his diminished financial standing, continued to be invited to friends' homes for dinner. He refused all invitations because he had always been able to arrive with a bottle of expensive wine under his arm; now he could not afford luxuries and he felt that to arrive without such a gift was socially unacceptable. He refused to recognize the fact that he was a desirable guest and that the invitations were extended not in the anticipation of getting a bottle of wine, but because of who he was.

Some of his lady friends continued to be interested in him. When he came to talk with me, one had been with him for more than a week but he was unable to have sexual intercourse with her. Despite their best efforts, his penis refused to cooperate and attain or maintain an erection. As Broderick has noted, "There is nothing more recalcitrant than a recalcitrant penis" (1978, p. 5). This man was frustrated, angry, feeling like a failure, and looking for a quick fix to his problem.

His doctor found no medical reason for his inability to achieve an erection. Obviously the problem was in his head, not in his body. Before he attempted to make love he would worry whether or not he would be able to get an erection, and if he had an erection, he worried whether he could maintain it. He tried to focus on amorous and sexual images and on his partner's body, but his mind always returned to his past failures. He was willing to admit that his business failure, his heart problems, and his reduced standard of living negatively influenced his feelings of self-esteem, but he could not afford the therapy that I recommended would help him move beyond his sexual problems. I never saw him again. I could only hope that in some moment of relaxation, perhaps after a good night's rest, he would discover that an erection and intercourse were possible.

YOU ARE NEVER TOO OLD

Whatever moral or ethical perspective one adopts, it is important to remember that elders are sexual beings. As the Penners note, we are all born male and female. Not all have the same innate bonding responses and not all are raised in environments where affection is displayed verbally or physically. Our sense of a sexual self responds to recognition. To be told that one looks beautiful, or that a new hair arrangement is attractive, or that a man's walk or stance is appreciated can only raise feelings of self-esteem. Elders in nursing homes respond to words of praise, to beauty parlor treatments for women and grooming exercises for men, to gestures and appropriate touching that express warmth and caring. The importance of appropriate touching has been emphasized over and over again in books directed toward the nursing profession. Touch breaks down barriers. Touch signifies acceptance. When elders feel that they have entered the social caste of the untouchables, in which expressions of caring and warmth are no longer appropriate or are considered undignified, the boundaries of existence become narrowed and the potential for expression of identity limited. Part of our identity is who we are sexually—man or woman, homosexual, heterosexual, or bisexual. Socially imposed limits to sexual expression constrict elders and smother spontaneous expressions of warmth and caring.

Elders are not "sexless" as some would label them. The greatest detriment to sexual fulfillment for most older women is the lack of sexual partners. There are no biological limits to their sexual capacity. Of course, as the body ages changes occur in some facets of sexuality. Menopause marks the end of potential child-bearing. For some women this introduces a time of new freedom in sexual enjoyment and activity—freedom from fears of pregnancy, from the need to use birth-control pills or contraceptive devices, from the nuisance of menstruation. For some women, there may be vaginal changes due to aging—greater difficulty in lubrication, a thinning of the vaginal walls which reduces the "cushioning effect" that may make some coital positions less comfortable, greater susceptibility to infection or inflammation caused by estrogen deficiency. Despite these potential problems, sexual desire, sexual capacity, and the potential for sexual enjoyment remain.

Sex can continue well into the ninth decade for healthy males. More time and more fondling of the sexual organs may be required to produce an erection. Because ejaculations do not occur as quickly as in youth, their female partners often enjoy greater satisfaction with multiple orgasms. The time between arousals may be longer. Sometimes the seminal fluid is thinner or the testes may be reduced in size. But these are minor problems. As I have written elsewhere, the greatest obstacles to sex for elders are the folktales pertaining to impotency, some religious taboos, and, most of all, the lack of opportunity (Larue 1983, p. 169). Broderick, commenting on the negative attitudes to elder sex, expressed his hopes for the future:

I am hopeful that, as we look at older people and their sexuality, our primary concern will be not only to treat them with dignity but also to permit them to be sexually attractive, to function as well as their circumstances will permit, and to encourage circumstances that do make it possible. More broadly, I hope we can make inputs into both the rising generation and the aging generation so that they can feel their own humanness, and their own sexuality as part of their humanness. (p. 8)

Elders do have sexual desires. They can and do make love. They enjoy and feel good about their sexual expressions. They find beauty in their bodies and in their expressions of love. There is nothing unwholesome, perverse, evil, or asocial in elder sexuality. Society has an ethical responsibility to respect and accept elder sexual needs and responses and to help older adults believe in themselves as whole persons. . Elders have the responsibility to reject agism and sexual stereotyping. If they want society to believe in them as whole persons, then they must have that faith in themselves. To ignore, denigrate, mock, or scorn elder sexuality is to reject, diminish and deny a part of their personalities and their humanness.

REFERENCES

Broderick, Carlfred. 1978. "Sexuality and Aging: An Overview," in Robert L. Solnick, ed. *Sexuality and Aging.* Los Angeles: University of Southern California Press, pp. 1-9.

Butler, Robert N., and Myrna I. Lewis. 1976. *Love and Sex After Sixty.* New York: Harper & Row.

Cooper, Thomas N. 1981. "Reactions of Staff to Sexuality of Nursing Home Patients," *Social Work* (November): 506-10.

Grotjahn, Martin. 1984. "Being Sick and Facing 80: Observations of an Aging Therapist," in Edwin S. Shneidman, ed., *Death: Current Perspectives,* 3d ed. Palo Alto, Calif.: Mayfield Publishing Company, pp. 249-57.

Hammond, Doris B. 1987. *My Parents Never Had Sex.* Buffalo, N.Y.: Prometheus Books.

Kaplan, Helen Singer. 1966. *Human Sexual Response.* Boston: Little, Brown and Company.

———. 1974. *The New Sex Therapy.* New York: Brunner/Mazel.

Larue, Gerald A. 1983. *Sex and the Bible.* Buffalo, N.Y.: Prometheus Books.

Miller, Dulcy B. 1978. "Sexual Practices and Administrative Policies in Long Term Care Institutions," in Robert L. Solnick, ed., *Sexuality and Aging*. Los Angeles: University of Southern California Press, pp. 163–75.

Penner, Clifford, and Joyce Penner. 1981. *The Gift of Sex: A Christian Guide to Sexual Fulfillment*. Dallas: Word Publishing.

Peterson, James A. 1968. *Married Love in the Middle Years*. New York: Association Press.

Pfeiffer, Eric. 1978. "Sexuality in the Aging Individual," in Robert L. Solnick, ed., *Sexuality and Aging*. Los Angeles: University of Southern California Press, pp. 26–32.

Starr, Bernard D., and Marcella Bakur Weiner. 1981. *The Starr-Weiner Report on Sex and Sexuality in the Mature Years*. New York: McGraw-Hill Book Company.

Steffl, Bernita M. 1978. "Sexuality and Aging: Implications for Nurses and Other Helping Professionals," in Robert L. Solnick, ed., *Sexuality and Aging*. Los Angeles: University of Southern California Press, pp. 132–53.

Sviland, Mary Ann P. 1978. "A Program of Sexual Liberation and Growth in the Elderly," in Robert L. Solnick, ed., *Sexuality and Aging*. Los Angeles: University of Southern California Press, pp. 96–114.

17

Elder Isolation and Loneliness

"It is not good for the man to be alone."

—Genesis 2:18

Loneliness, according to one definition, "is a response to the quantity and quality of one's social life" (Perlman 1982, p. 333). These feelings reflect a deficiency in relationships growing out of loss (whether it be income, employment, possessions, close friends, spouses, or the like) isolation, depression, and grief. Perhaps most elders experience only temporary loneliness, for others the phenomenon is pervasive.

Happily married elders are able to share memories, interests, problems, concerns, and intimacy; unhappily married elders, the widowed, and the single are compelled to find confidants and companionship elsewhere. Perlman cites a 1976 San Francisco research project demonstrating that "intimacy and the capacity for mutuality are vital factors in the well-being of older adults." At the same time, the study showed that "contact with kin does not reduce loneliness and enhance psychological well-being among older adults, while contact with peers often does" (1982, p. 334). No one would suggest that social interaction with family members is unimportant. But some family relationships are built on feelings of "ought" or obligation, rather than on personal desire and enjoyment of sharing; others, while satisfying, have never been open to intimate discussion. Elders benefit by association with nonfamily members when the relationship is based on shared interests and mutuality. Friends and confidants are contributors to mental and physical health and are barriers to loneliness.

CAUSES OF LONELINESS

Some elders make and keep friends easily; for others the process is difficult. Trustworthiness and reliability are basic to healthy relationships. Experience and training have made some elderly persons suspicious of others and unwilling to trust. Some are shy and hesitate to telephone or write to friends; they suffer the restrictions of self-imposed protocols that inhibit spontaneity in reaching out. It is important for mental and physical health for an elder to know that someone—a friend or family member—is available and can be counted on to respond when needed. Responses made on a hit-or-miss basis engender distrust of one's ability to make reliable friends. This leads to destructive feelings of depression and helplessness (Seligman 1975).

Some elders become so reliant on a small circle of friends and confidants that when these persons die or relocate, loneliness ensues, often accompanied by feelings that there can be no replacements. Unlike the young, for whom life appears to represent a continuing adventurous exploration of new encounters, new associations, and new friendships, for many elders, life is experienced as a shrinking of relationships and of opportunities to meet new people.

As we have noted, for some elders retirement constitutes the ultimate loss of one's role in society. Occupational involvement is the foundation upon which they have built personal and social identity plus a great deal of meaning in life. Friends and companions were fellow workers and their families. With retirement, relationships to the familiar work force have altered; the retiree becomes a "has-been" and the person's input is no longer accepted or respected.

Role changes in family relations are also part of the elder experience. Bonding differs from family to family. In some settings, the relationship between parent and child is so very close that there is daily contact by visits or telephone. When such intimate contact is possible, elders tend not to feel isolated or abandoned.

Familial distancing may begin when children leave home for college; in a separate and away-from-home environment, they begin to develop their unique identities. They may meet the person they will someday marry— someone who is not the boy or girl next door. The partner-to-be is a stranger with a family of his or her own and with a background and interests that are foreign to the elders. Marriage increases children's independence. Many offspring become industrial migrants who follow promotions and job potentials wherever they may be found. In distant cities, they form new friendships and create their own unique familial and social environment. Where familial bonding and dependent relationships are strong and demanding, closeness is maintained by telephone calls and constant letter writing. Where the bonds are looser, contact is infrequent and often superficial. Meanwhile, the elders enter forced retirement and feel functionless and isolated from the money-producing world and from their children, who are part of that active, involved world.

Elders tend to be most comfortable with the lifestyle they have developed over years of living together. Their children, in a new family setting, produce different living and thinking patterns. Visits can be difficult, strained, marked with patient or impatient toleration of, what in the children's eyes are, the elders' hardened, fixed beliefs and, what to the elders appears as, the radical or challenging attitudes of the children. When families live near to one another the changes do not seem so dramatic. When distances are great and visits are rare, differences in family patterns can be upsetting. Elders may feel estranged. Their children are different, changed and distant. They appear to have abandoned what the elders may have considered established patterns or values.

On the other hand, there are instances where the elders remain flexible and open to growth, while the offspring move into adamant, fixed, and unyielding positions. Such situations often occur when children become attached to some religious group with closed, separatist, and exclusionary beliefs or get caught up in some far-fetched mystical craze, such as belief in the magic of crystals, or become devotees of astrology or followers of some so-called psychic leader (see Larue 1990). Elders, who have watched such faddish notions come and go, may feel that their children have abandoned reason; they may question the wisdom, if not the sanity, of these younger family members. To avoid the isolation that emerges from the development of different life patterns, elders and children must learn either to tolerate one another's differences or to remain silent about their own commitments, disappointments, and feelings of estrangement—and this is not always easy to do.

When family businesses are passed on to offspring, problems may develop with the elders' inability to let go. Consider the case of a mom-and-pop business that, over the years, develops into a healthy organization yielding profits that enable the elders to retire in comfort. The company is taken over and slowly bought out by the eldest daughter. The elders establish a new home about one hundred miles from the business. On those occasions when the elders visit with the daughter at the business site, quarrels erupt over company policy and the way to run the enterprise.

The elders feel angry and rejected; they think the daughter has become hard-nosed and intolerant. Their ideas, once appreciated and acted upon, are now debated and treated as intrusions. Their life in retirement has become functionless, meaningless. They feel isolated from family and from the business world.

Feelings of isolation may also result from spousal death. The loss of a companion of many years, with whom one has shared both good and bad times, can be overwhelming. Often this loss is accompanied by depression, grief, guilt, feelings of emptiness, and unbelievable loneliness. Coping with such feelings will be discussed below.

Elders can be lonely in institutional settings. Discrimination based on differences can subtly isolate an individual. Race, creed, color, and political affiliations are the most familiar bases for distancing. Physical handicaps, deformities, and speech impediments following strokes can motivate both staff and residents to avoid social contact. The afflicted person is shunted off into a corner, so to speak, receiving, to all appearances, regular care, but suffering the sense of being shunned.

CONFRONTING LONELINESS

Loneliness is not the equivalent of being alone. One can be alone and not be lonely, just as one can be in a crowd of people and be lonely. Aloneness is a state of being; loneliness is a response. Gene has been a bachelor all of his life. He is sixty-five years of age, retired, and lives alone. He has friends who range in age from a six-year-old neighbor child who considers him a second grandpa, to men and women he has worked with over the years. He is active and involved in social issues and events. He is alone much of the time, just as he has been throughout his life, but he is not lonely.

Elizabeth, on the other hand, experiences loneliness. Her husband of forty-six years died a year ago. They had shared every trial, every tribulation, every success and every joy throughout their marriage. When her hearing failed and she could no longer hear the telephone ring, her husband installed a flashing light and an amplified receiver on the phone. Should she not see the light flash, he would call her attention to it. They shopped, gardened, watched television together, and talked over life's events. Elizabeth has friends and family who spend time with her. She can handle being alone, because she has been alone in silence with her deafness for many years, but she is also lonely because she misses her lifelong companion.

Abject loneliness is something quite different. It involves feelings of separation and isolation, of having no meaningful relationships (Potthoff 1976, p. 11). Loneliness that results from social and economic situations differs from that caused by personal factors. After the death of her husband, an elderly woman who lived in a small town where she had spent her entire life was persuaded by her family to sell the family home and move to a large city where she would be closer to her children. She purchased a two-room suite in a retirement home, moved in some of her cherished furniture (the rest was sold or given away) and found herself depressed, lonely, and lost. Her children phoned each day and visited her about once a week. She was terrified by the hugeness of the city and she had no transportation. The food in the residential setting was not what she was used to and she knew no one there in the intimate, caring way she had known friends in her home town. In her loneliness, she spent hours reviewing family albums and just sitting—dozing and dreaming. She seldom walked, because there was no place to go except to a local shopping mall, and she tired of watching other people interrelate while she sat alone as an outside observer. She began to dwell more and more in the past. When her family came to visit and take her out on weekends, they were convinced that she was becoming senile. She had no one to tell her who she was by relating to her as a significant other. The staff at the residence were business-like and responsible to dozens of other elders; they simply could not and would not take the time to visit with her. She felt trapped in an isolated and meaningless life.

It was pointless to argue that there was still a great deal of living to be done. She would shrug and ask, "Where?" She missed the familiar intimacy of her large old home, the nearby church, and her acceptance by a congregation of families with whom she had grown up. Coming to the city was a mistake. She had acted too quickly out of her grief; counted on her busy, involved offspring to replace the mate she had lost; and expected them to provide a new social environment in which she could feel that she belonged. Now she felt that she was a burden to everyone, including herself.

It is not surprising to find that there are many therapists who are convinced that loneliness contributes to poor health and suicide. Indeed, it is not uncommon for many days to pass before the body of an elder who dies in isolation is discovered. The idea of neighborhood has faded. Now many elders live in apartment complexes with hundreds of units. In these structures composed of separate cells, few know or care who lives above or below them, next door or across the hall.

Loneliness may develop when a spouse becomes afflicted with Alzheimer's Disease and can no longer be a companion, friend, or lover. When the ailing spouse is institutionalized, the aloneness of the healthy spouse can be relieved by involvement in extramarital relationships. Letters to "Dear Abby" which appeared in the *Los Angeles Times,* September 3, 1990, and which Ms. Van Buren has graciously permitted me to reproduce, point to the ethical dilemma.

> Dear Abby: My wife has had Alzheimer's for several years and is now totally bedridden. She doesn't even recognize me. My life has been very lonely. My children have encouraged me to get out and enjoy the last years of my life. (I am 73 and my wife is 75.)
>
> To get to the point, I started seeing a 68-year-old widow who lives in my condo complex. We go to dinner, theater, concerts. We are good company for each other, but the flak we are getting from some of our neighbors is very upsetting.
>
> What is your opinion of this? Do I have the right to enjoy my life? And what about the woman I'm seeing? Does she have the right to date me—a married man?
>
> —Single, But Not Single

> Dear Single, But: Since there is no hope for your wife's recovery, and she no longer recognizes you, I see no reason why you and your neighbor can't enjoy each other's company. Easing the burden of loneliness isn't desertion, so don't allow anyone to lay a guilt trip on you. Read on for the flip side of your situation.

> Dear Abby: Dad died suddenly of a massive heart attack on the tennis court. It was a terrible shock to Mom. They had been married for 48 years.
>
> Mom's New Age therapist gave her one year only to mourn Dad's death, then she *ordered* her to get on with her life. This therapist then introduced Mom to an older man whom she had been treating for depression. The man's wife has Alzheimer's and has been out of touch with reality for many years.
>
> You can probably guess the rest of this story. Now Mom, at age 70, is keeping company with this married man. (She says it's platonic, but I'm not so sure.) I've been trying to persuade her to break it off with him. My two brothers see nothing wrong with her conduct and tell me to mind my business.
>
> How do you see it, Abby? Isn't a man whose wife has an incurable illness considered married? Whatever happened to "for better or worse, in sickness and in health—till death do us part"?
>
> Geraldine (Not My Real Name)

Dear Geraldine: Of course the man is "still married," but his wife is living somewhere between heaven and Earth, and the likelihood of her returning is nil. If your mother says their relationship is platonic, why not believe her?

To answer your question: If I were terminally ill with no chance of recovery and no longer recognized my husband, I would want him to live the remainder of his life with as much happiness as possible. And I would hope that the community would treat him with understanding and compassion—and not rush to judgment.

THE FEAR OF LONELINESS

A fear of loneliness is often expressed by isolated elders who live alone. They fear being injured within their living quarters and unable to summon help. One lonely Elder put his fears this way: "I could be dying or dead for several days in my apartment and no one would know. No one would miss me. Finally, someone would call and get no answer and perhaps investigate. In the long run, the smell of my decaying body would probably offend the neighbors and they would ask for an investigation!" Presently various forms of "Medic Alert" are available. The injured elder need only push a button on a small instrument worn on a chain around the neck to summon help.

Others fear disorientation that grows out of lack of contact with other human beings. Nursing home personnel have remarked on the rapid decline in mental functioning of residents who feel abandoned by family and, despite the presence of staff and other residents, lonely and insecure. As one staff person remarked, "Either they have the will to adapt and pull out of the depression or they sink into some kind of senility."

An all-night talk-show host commented, "the dark hours after midnight are the loneliest hours of all" (Mark 1978, p. 18). It was then that isolated individuals used the open lines of the talk-show to make contact with another human being, to share ideas and to engage in dialogue. It was also then that the talk-show host would receive calls from lonely and suicidal persons, which he took on private rather than public phone lines.

COPING WITH LONELINESS

Coping has to begin with the individual. There are outside resources that can help, but the lonely individual must take the steps to deal with his or her feelings.

In the gathering-in-the-home after a funeral, the daughter of the sixty-five-year-old widow asked me, "Will all these people be available to help my mother deal with her grief?" The daughter lived in another city and would soon return to her own family and employment. I was honest. "No, these people have their own lives to live and their own responsibilities. Some will phone. Some will visit. But many were friends of your father through his work. Your mother is going to have to find her own way." It was not a pleasant answer, but it was honest. Eventually, the mother, who had inner strengths perhaps unknown to the daughter, did work through her grief and "got on with" her life.

"Grief work" is "a term coined by Sigmund Freud for the process of disengagement from the lost person that bereaved people must go through if they are to make a healthy recovery" (McConnell and Anderson 1980, p. 11). The term can be applied to the necessary coping pattern elders must experience for any loss including loss of work through retirement, loss of a child, loss of income, loss of health, and, most of all, loss of a spouse (see chapter 19). It suggests that the steps may not be easy; recovery involves work—doing something to bring healing.

Any loss produces shock to the system, but some losses provoke anger —particularly those associated with forced retirement. Something important is being taken away. The isolation from the familiar can develop into depression, which Freud has told us is anger turned inward. Self-blame and feelings of inability to cope deepen the depression and reinforce the sense of being isolated. It is important that the elder recognize these emotions as legitimate, but not binding. At this point, recovery depends on the elder's ability to take charge of his or her life and to move beyond self-deprecation, anger, and isolation.

As the widowed woman began to work through her grief, she assessed her feelings. When the forced retiree moved beyond his anger, he evaluated his potential. Like every other lonely elder, each had to reach deep inside of the self to discover resources that could be tapped. All such probing must begin with an analysis of what is taking place now, with a candid look at one's emotional responses and at what these feelings are doing to the person. Sometimes therapeutic help is required and it is vital that community services have provisions for elder counseling. University and college psychology and counseling programs often provide free or low-cost therapeutic treatment by supervised student interns. Many elders receive help from such programs; others claim that the youthful counselors lack the experience, the insight, or the understanding of the elder world to provide much help. They may know the theories, but they cannot grasp the many facets of elder life and the emotional pain older adults feel. Social service agencies provide counseling but are often so overburdened that they lack resources to provide the therapy so essential to elder adjustment to both change and loneliness. They may suggest things that these older persons can do, but helping an elder to cope with loneliness calls for something more than a list of "ought tos" or "why dontchas."

Peer group sessions led by a trained counselor can be helpful. Here elders discover that they are not the only ones to experience loneliness. Sharing feelings and hearing how others cope can lift the spirit.

It has often been pointed out that just as thoughts can influence how one feels—that is, the mind leads the body—so, too, can the body lead the mind. Physical exercise, which may be nothing more than a long walk, can give a powerful lift to depressed feelings and may help motivate the elder to take charge of the loneliness. If the elder has his or her own home, garden work can buoy up spirits.

For elders who find opportunity for employment, retirement does not signify the abandonment of a life of active earning and respected contribution. The importance of work involvement was clearly stated in the words of a former bank vice president. Each time we would meet he would assure me, "I am gainfully employed." But he was never really happy away from his life's work. When he and his wife traveled abroad, she would visit art galleries and archaeological sites; he headed for the nearest bank where he could talk with persons who shared his fascination with finance. Although he had always seemed to be in good health, he died three years after his forced retirement. It was as if he had become spiritually isolated when the work that gave meaning to his life was taken from him.

Some elders engage in volunteer work, where their contribution of energy and time are appreciated. Often the tasks they are assigned are important but menial. A woman who formerly managed a busy office finds herself stuffing envelopes to be mailed in an appeal for funds. She feels her skills are not appreciated. Her experience as a trained and capable manager has been negated and the volunteer assignment appears trivial to her. Inwardly, she has not relinquished her earlier role. She would feel appreciated if her volunteer activities placed her in a challenging position where new dimensions of work related to her background and training called for effort and growth. In other words, meaning-filled post-retirement activities are those that continue the process of role exit and role advancement normally experienced throughout life. Organizations that welcome elders as volunteers can contribute to feelings of isolation by their indirect lack of appreciation and by failing to use elder talents and skills.

Neighborhood centers where young and old gather, churches and other social groups that bring elders together, make important contributions to helping the elderly overcome feelings of isolation and loneliness. Some elders refuse to limit association to their own age group. They give time and energy to involvement in university, college, and high-school activities that provide interaction with youth and emerging social changes. My gerontology classes are open to elders who enroll as auditors (they are not interested in grades) and who contribute and enrich discussions because of their personal backgrounds and experiences.

Poor health can contribute to loneliness. This often leads to housebound elders becoming dependent on outsiders for visits. One elder uses the long hours when she is alone to write letters to friends and relatives. Her mail box is always filled with responses. She has learned to write whether or not the person responds and her loneliness is alleviated by letters and by phone calls from those with whom she corresponds. She has evaluated her situation and has taken action to alleviate her loneliness. As a by-product of her letter writing, those to whom she writes often visit when they are in her city. Her home is open. She keeps a supply of cookies and easily prepared food in her deep freezer. She has a spare bedroom that visitors can occupy. This woman has responded positively and creatively to a negative life setting.

Elders who are patients in nursing homes cannot exercise the same kind of controls over their situation as those who are free to move about and set their own schedules. Some, who are isolated in their individual rooms, need more human contact to alleviate loneliness than association with busy staff personnel. Mobile residents can alleviate their own and others' loneliness by visiting with other patients, particularly with those who cannot move about freely. Through sharing time and by helping others they contribute to their own need to be useful and involved. Volunteer visitors, who are free to spend time talking, touching, sharing, provide residents with a breath of fresh air through their willingness to give personal attention to disabled elders.

The loneliness of others motivates the caring human to reach out to alleviate the isolation of others, but in reaching out there can be risks to personal privacy. One family learned of a lonely elder who had attempted suicide, so they invited the woman to their home for Sunday dinner. Soon the shared Sunday dinner became a regular event. She began to arrive earlier and earlier and stay later and later. She watched television with the family, often insisting that they tune in her favorite programs. Soon she was at the door in late afternoons on days other than Sunday, and, of course, was invited to stay for dinner. When the family went on outings, she was included, but mostly out of politeness. The couple's children complained about the invasion of privacy and the parents finally acknowledged that their efforts to entertain this particular elder had gone beyond their intentions. But how could they now impose limits on an established pattern? They finally had to assert their wishes. The elder was angry and hurt, but she had to make choices—recognize the legitimacy of the complaints and comply with the new regulations or lose the benefits of this helpful and health-giving association. She chose the former. The caring family now felt comfortable with her presence. They could invite or not invite her to some gatherings. She assumed the role of "special friend" rather than that of "family member" (which she would have preferred). Her case became a model for others who were interested in reaching out to lonely elders. The rule here for caregivers is: after the initial contacts, if the elder is one who can be welcomed into the home as a visitor, open the door to more associations, but set the limits in clear and understandable terms that do not fluctuate.

Some elders alleviate their own sense of isolation by developing entertainment patterns with others in their age group. They meet on given days in one another's living quarters to talk, to exchange ideas, to play cards, to share memories, and to establish friendships. Once again, elders help elders cope with loneliness.

It is not surprising to find that some older adults need more than social gatherings and activities to alleviate loneliness. They find someone to marry. One university researcher, just past eighty years of age and still involved in his important work, married a family friend who was sixty-three years of age, just one year after his wife's death. "I am tired of living alone," he said, "and she is too." Like others who find themselves alone and aged, they assuaged loneliness with new, intimate companionship.

We all have social responsibilities, but the first obligation must be to ourselves. As much as possible, each elder has a duty to act in ways that enhance the self by responding to personal feelings of isolation and loneliness. The second obligation is to others. Each caring person can reach out to those who need human contact to maintain their stability in times of loneliness. In the complexity of modern society, the tendency has been to place the obligation of caring for isolated others on institutions rather than on individuals. Nevertheless, the capacity to experience empathy is still a vital part of our humanity and our humanness. The courage to act on those feelings, to risk being a friend to a lonely elder, constitutes an ethical response that can only be ignored at the risk of denying an integral part of our social awareness and responsibility.

REFERENCES

Burnside, I. 1971. "Loneliness in Old Age," *Mental Hygiene* 55, pp. 391–97.

Kohn, Jane Burgess, and Willard K. Burgess. 1978. *The Widower*. Boston: Beacon Press.

Larue, Gerald A. 1990. *The Supernatural, the Occult, and the Bible*. Buffalo, N.Y.: Prometheus Books.

Lee, Gary R., and Masako Ishii-Kuntz. 1987. "Social Interaction, Loneliness, and Emotional Well-Being Among the Elderly," *Research in Aging* 9, No. 4 (December): 459–82.

Lynch, James J. 1977. *The Broken Heart: The Medical Consequences of Loneliness*. New York: Basic Books, Inc.

Mark, Norman. 1978. "Loneliness: The Me Nobody Knows," *The Los Angeles Times,* December 3, pp. 18–20.

McConnell, Adeline, and Beverly Anderson. 1980. *Single After Fifty*. New York: McGraw-Hill.

Natale, Samuel M. 1986. "Loneliness and the Aging Client: Psychotherapeutic Considerations," in Samuel M. Natale, ed., *Psychotherapy and the Lonely Patient*. New York: Haworth Press.

Perlman, P. 1982. *Loneliness*. New York: Wiley-Interscience Publications.

Potthoff, Harvey H. 1976. *Loneliness: Understanding and Dealing With It*. Nashville, Tenn.: Abingdon. (Paperback edition by Harper and Row, New York, titled *Understanding Loneliness,* 1977.)

Ryan, Maura C., and Joanne Petterson. "Loneliness in the Elderly," *Journal of Gerontological Nursing* 13, no. 5, pp. 6–11.

Seligman, Martin E. R. 1975. *Helplessness*. San Francisco: W. H. Freeman and Company.

18

Elder Courage

"To be or not to be, that is the question."

—Shakespeare, *Hamlet*

Courage, according to Rollo May, is not to be understood as the opposite of despair but rather "the capacity to move ahead *in spite of despair.*" (1975, p. 3).* This kind of courage is not to be confused with rashness, bravado, or stubbornness but "requires a centeredness within our own being, without which we would feel ourselves to be a vacuum" (ibid.). Many elders express this kind of courage, which embraces the physical, the moral/ethical, and the social dimensions of existence. They confront with courage the fears associated with aging—fears of loneliness, of abandonment, of poverty, of infirmity, of dying, and of death.

THE ABILITY TO ADAPT

One of the silliest aphorisms applied to elders is "You can't teach an old dog new tricks." In the first place, elders are not dogs; in the second place, the learning capacity and the ability to adapt that characterizes elder lifestyles demonstrates the absurdity of this outmoded saying. Elders can and do learn new tricks!

Elder courage is reflected in an ability to adapt that enables personal and social change and growth to take place. Elder adaptability can be

---

*The emphasis here is May's.

217

immediately appreciated in view of the description of the dramatic social and technological changes that have occurred during their lifetime. As we have noted, from radios to television, from woodburning stoves to microwaves, from canning fruits for the winter to frozen vegetables, from washboards to electric washers and dryers, elders have, like well-rooted willows, swayed with the winds of change and remained anchored in who and what they are.

Changing social patterns have not fazed elders for they have been part of the change. They flowed with the migration from the farm to the city, the growth of the town into the city and the city into the megalopolis. They have lived through wars; depressions; unemployment; inflation; radical social changes (e.g., voter rights for women and Prohibition); racial, religious, and political bigotry; and the emancipation of women, races, and other minorities. Many were actively involved in the dramatic social shifts and conflicts. They have experienced a variety of destructive losses ranging from friends and family members through death or separation by distance, to possessions through the effects of storms, floods, earthquakes, fires, and theft, to the personal ravages of ailments associated with aging including arthritis, rheumatism, heart or lung impairment, and so forth. Throughout their lives, the elderly have survived a number of major medical emergencies: polio, tuberculosis, and the typhoid fever epidemic, all of which are now virtually eradicated (though tuberculosis now seems to be attempting a comeback). Through adaptation they have survived to confront each new circumstance.

Now, having become elders, they reveal the capacity for continuing adaptation. Even the 5 percent or so of elders who are confined to nursing homes and long-term care facilities reveal an amazing ability to adapt whenever they are given the opportunity. The greater the amount of freedom for personal expression and development that such institutions provide, the more the creative adaptability of the elder is manifested. Those institutions that restrict the mobility of elders by presenting as the central meeting place nonactive sitting facilities such as television rooms only serve to stifle growth. Facilities that rely on sedation to keep elders quiet and conforming reduce the potential for involvement in health-preserving responses ranging from intellectual exchange of opinions and ideas to physical activity that enhances feelings of well-being. On the other hand, institutions that through organization of space and facilities maximize the ability of elders to experience freedom of choice in activities, movement and personal time arrangements encourage continuing participation in the world of ideas and action that have long been a part of the elder's history.

CONCERNING COURAGE

What is equally important is the recognition of personal or individual elder courage. It is no small matter to witness the shrinkage of the world in which one has been active. The ability of elders to be on their own despite physical handicaps can only continue to amaze.

Here is a well-educated eighty-year-old woman who despite her frailty continues to involve herself in social action projects. Her life is characterized by a continuing list of personal losses. She had been an actress, involved with people, roles, causes, and with the freedom to pursue her own course. Little by little, her choices have become increasingly limited by one physical ailment after another. Today, she hobbles around with a walker, depends on a friend to drive her to meetings, and despite the crippling effects of arthritis in her hands she still manages to type and write letters and articles for publication. She speaks frequently to local societies and uses the telephone to reach out to the world she cannot visit. It is not easy, she admits, but what are her alternatives? She resents the ravages of age that compel her to depend on others and that limit her potential; but despite the pain and the limitations she remains active. Her courage falters at only one point—the thought of experiencing the same kind of "fate" that accompanied her sisters before they died. They spent their last years in failing health in nursing homes, confined to an institution, completely dependent on others. She will not go that route. She does not want someone to change diapers for her, bathe her, dress her, walk her like a puppy. She has plans for the ending of her life should her last days begin to parallel those of her sisters. And this decision can also be understood as an act of courage. She will be in charge of her own life and of her own death.

Courage to confront life despite limiting and irritating handicaps is characteristic of elders. Most refuse to quit or give up. They struggle for independence and seem only to lose something of the spark of living when they are forced to become completely dependent upon others. The last choice open to them is that of suicide.

THE COURAGE NOT TO BE

The number of elders taking their own lives is on the increase. White males kill themselves more often than white females, black males, or black females (Eddy and Alles 1983, pp. 165f). The causes for elder suicide vary but they are often associated with loss of status, position, power, and money. As the social world of the elder shrinks through the death of peers and through personal incapacitation, the quality of life diminishes and questions of personal worth surface. Feelings of loneliness, depression, despair, and of being unloved and unlovable grow out of isolation. The death of a spouse may increase the feelings of isolation and loneliness and lead to suicide. Depression and despair with the accompanying feeling of helplessness can be contributing factors. Some depression can be related to alcoholism or to the overuse of prescribed drugs that produce depression as a side-effect. Chronic disease and the diagnosis of terminal illness can also trigger feelings of depression. For elders who are trapped in these destructive moods suicide becomes an acceptable response.

IS ELDER SUICIDE IMMORAL?

Most discussions about the morality of self-killing deal with suicide in general, which is to say that the focus is not simply on elders. Suicide prevention centers and suicide hotlines are confronted daily with younger persons who contemplate taking their own lives because of failure in love, marriage, business, school, relationships, family, and so on. Counselors seek to deter the act and help the individual discover that his or her particular life is worth preserving and that there are acceptable and workable alternatives to suicide.

Some religious groups oppose suicide. They argue that life is a gift of God and only He should determine when that life should end—not humans. Theological condemnations of suicide are often based on the kind of reasoning found in the writings of Thomas Aquinas (e.g., the *Summa Theologica*). He based his objections and his classification of suicide as a sin in part on biblical texts, including the commandment "Thou shalt not kill" (fifth in Roman Catholic listings, sixth in Protestant codes) and on the following statement attributed to God: "I will kill and I will make to live" (Deut. 32:39). Aquinas argued that life was a divine gift and subject to divine power, therefore the suicidal person sins against God just as if the person were to kill another person's slave. Drawing upon Aristotle's *Nicomachean Ethics,* he stated that self-killing deprived the community of which the individual was a part. He believed that taking life was contrary to nature (Donnelly 1990, p. 34).

Under ordinary circumstances, one might agree with some aspects of Aquinas's reasoning. Most life is geared to self-preservation, and in many instances a death does deprive a community of strength. But for frail, helpless, dependent, ailing elders these arguments hold no meaning. Life has run its course and one can only agree with David Hume: "That suicide may often be consistent with interest and with our duty to ourselves, no one can question, who allows that age, sickness or misfortune, may render life a burden, and make it worse even than annihilation" (Donnelly 1990, p. 44). As to the deprivation of society, elders can argue that by taking their own lives they remove a burden from society, thus relieving others of the need to expend time and money for their continuing care. Elders are aware that in the eyes of some they are a social burden, and that very idea negates any feelings they have of worth and dignity.

So far as the importance and validity of religious arguments are concerned, individuals can only decide for themselves (see Larue 1985). In the past some religious groups denied suicides the right to be buried in sacred ground and even the services of the church; today most enlightened clergy treat the act with compassion and focus on the spiritual and emotional needs of the family.

Obviously there are situations that appear to make committing suicide seem both rational and appropriate. A person, utterly alone, miserable, and in fear of dying a long and painful death may reason that to terminate life before it gets any worse is a most appropriate choice. After all, why should a person be compelled to continue to live a rapidly decaying life? Another, having experienced the feelings of pain and helplessness when a loved one died after being hooked up to a respirator and to life-supporting machines, may decide that rather than being put through such indignities immediate death would relieve significant friends and family of the kind of pain and suffering he or she experienced with a loved one. In other words, there are situations where the decision to commit suicide can be understood as reasonable and appropriate.

Perhaps the greatest social concern in admitting the right of elders to take their own lives is that public acceptance of the act might prompt a rash of such suicides including some who have much to contribute to life. In other words, elders might abandon the principle of courage that enables heroic coping with life and opt for suicide, which symbolizes giving up on life. Some might be led to believe that suicide is obligatory for all frail or failing elders.

Years ago, I was a guest of those charged with administering a home for retired screen actors. An elderly actress had just taken her own life. The staff decided not to tell the residents what had occurred because they feared that other frail elders might emulate her act. At this point it became obvious that the staff did not trust the residents' ability to handle the actress' chosen means of dying. What these younger staff persons ignored was the fact that resident elders had confronted deaths of friends and relatives over and over again during their lifetimes and that suicide was not unknown in the acting profession. I felt confident that the elders could handle the fact and that they had the right to know and not be treated like fragile, impressionable children. In other words, I believe that residents had the courage to continue to live despite the example set by a friend, and that they would not think that because she had taken her life they were obligated to do the same.

I couldn't view the actress' suicide as an act of cowardice. Although choosing to live in difficult circumstances is recognized as an act of courage, the taking of one's own life despite the natural urge to survive is equally an act of courage. With an elder, such a choice usually grows out of reflection and is unlike the spur-of-the-moment reaction to anguish that is so characteristic of youthful suicide. The act reflects the experience of emptiness or of lack of meaning—the sense that life, as it is being experienced, is devoid of worth. One could challenge this response on the basis of the sentiments expressed in the Frank Capra film *It's a Wonderful Life,* in which the character George Bailey (played by Jimmy Stewart), having been rescued from a suicide, is given an opportunity to review his life to discover what his presence has meant both directly and indirectly to a multitude of people. But for the aging actress, the past was the past; it was the present that was devoid of significance and purpose. She chose not to live in such a situation, and her choice can be recognized as an act of personal courage.

Just as the notion of suicide as a sin has been quietly set aside in most religions, so can the claim that the self-killing by an elder results in social loss. The tremendous drain on finances, time, energy, and so forth expended on the care of an elder for whom the quality of life has deteriorated and who has no desire to live, can be alleviated by the elder's choice of death. This person's suicide could be interpreted as a beneficent social act.

What does remain as an ethical issue is the potential pain to be borne by survivors. As with the death of any significant other, feelings of loss, separation, and anguish can result from elder suicide. On the other hand, in case after case, I have been told of the mixed emotions of grief and relief that such deaths have engendered. The grief is the normal response to loss; the relief is the normal response to the termination of the elder's unhappy existence. If the elder has made closure—if proper farewells and expressions of love and caring have been made—the grief reactions are abated. Sometimes feelings of guilt surface: the living should have been more aware and more responsive to the elder's despondency. This guilt may be valid because, as we shall see, despondency and loneliness are contributing factors in some elder suicides—factors that can be alleviated by caregivers, friends, and relatives.

Elders who contemplate suicide must, of necessity, exercise caution in sharing their intentions because well-meaning friends and relatives need only to make a report to the police or social service agencies to initiate intervention procedures. Caring and sensitive elders can ease the burdens of their suicides by leaving farewell letters or tape recordings expressing love and instructions concerning the disposal of the body. Wills that make explicit the disposal of possessions can alleviate the confusion that often follows suicidal death. If elder suicide can be recognized as an ethical choice, then the person contemplating suicide has the moral responsibility to do everything in his or her power to make the death as painless as possible for survivors.

Elder suicide is on the rise. Ann Wickett's studies demonstrated that whereas only three double suicides were recorded in the 1970s, thirty-one were reported in the 1980s. One can surmise that if the pattern continues, more will take place in the 1990s.

Suicide is by no means a necessary or desirable step for most elders. Society in general and families in particular need to recognize that much can be done to alleviate the negative feelings that lead to self-destruction. Supportive services that keep the elder functioning are very important. Chores that drain energy and seem to be overwhelming for frail elders can be handled by visiting domestic assistants and, at times, by family members. Clinical health services that provide counseling for the depressed elder, geriatric day-care, and outpatient supports do much to keep the elder spirits from flagging. In time of crisis and need, elder suicide can be prevented by supportive services.

Unfortunately not many persons are trained to recognize the signs of impending suicide. If there is genuine ethical concern about elder suicide, then the elderly and those who work with them and, indeed, the public at large, need to be made aware of the signs and symptoms of depression that can lead to suicide and be informed of ways to prevent self-killing.

What are the signs of impending suicide? They include both forthright and subtle statements such as "Life has no meaning for me," "I won't be troubling you anymore," or "I feel I can't go on." Often these statements are met with denial: "Oh, come now, you mustn't talk like that!" or "Stop this silly talk!" or "You've got many more years ahead of you." An elder may suddenly begin to dispose of treasured belongings saying, "I don't need them any longer." Unless the recipient asks why, it is often assumed that the elder has grown beyond these items; the real reason never surfaces.

An elder who has been depressed for a long time suddenly becomes very active and involved in cleaning up living quarters, writing letters to friends, making a will, all the while smiling or expressing cheer. The "smiling depressive" is one of the most deceptive of potential suicides. The smile often means they have a plan in mind and they know what they are going to do to end their inner agony. To the outsider, these elders seem to have moved away from depression when quite the opposite is the case.

The clues are often there; they need to be recognized. Once the words are understood, the door is opened for conversation in depth. What lies behind the feeling of need to kill oneself? Are there alternative choices? Out of the discussion may come an understanding of what the elder is feeling and either what can be done to help meet the needs or, on the other hand, a deep appreciation of what the elder intends to do.

THE COURAGE TO BE

Of course, because one is suffering the pains and limitations often associated with aging, one need not choose death. Viktor E. Frankl (1963), out of his Nazi concentration camp experiences, found meaning in suffering and was impressed by the courage of those who survived the ordeal by focussing on the opportunities in their present horrible situation. The setting required "a fundamental change in our attitude toward life" (p. 122). The concern was not an effort to find meaning in life but in adapting to where they were in life. "When a man finds that it is his destiny to suffer, he will have to accept his destiny as his task; his single and unique task. He will have to acknowledge the fact that even in suffering he is unique and alone in the universe. No one can relieve him of his suffering or suffer in his place. His unique opportunity lies in the way in which he bears his burden" (Frankl 1963, pp. 123–24). Individuals were free to choose the ways in which they confronted life.

> A man who let himself decline because he could not see any future goal found himself occupied with retrospective thoughts. In a different connection, we have already spoken of the tendency there was to look into the past, to help make the present, with all its horrors, less real.

But in robbing the present of its reality there lay a certain danger. It became easy to overlook the opportunities to make something positive of camp life, opportunities which really did exist. Regarding our "provisional existence" as unreal was in itself an important factor in causing prisoners to lose their hold on life; everything in a way became pointless. Such people forgot that often it is just such an exceptionally difficult external situation which gives man an opportunity to grow spiritually beyond himself. Instead of taking the camp's difficulties as a test of their inner strength, they did not take their life seriously and despised it as something of no consequence. They preferred to close their eyes and live in the past. Life for such people became meaningless. (Frankl 1963, pp. 113–14)

The courage to continue to exist despite suffering and the horror of subsistence in a concentration camp became a matter of choice linked to the belief that the individual had unfinished business in life. Clearly, to find meaning in such a setting is testimony to the human courage to be.

In a public meeting, after a discussion on meaning in life, a sixty-eight-year-old man in quiet tones, said, "I hate myself. I have always hated myself. It is not that I am a homosexual, it is just that I don't like who I am. I have no friends. People in the mobile home park where I live, ignore me. I am alone and I hate myself." There was no opportunity to explore in depth the basis for his reactions (see chapter 10), but he came across as a pleasant, helpful, concerned, articulate human being. I had watched him help in the arrangement of chairs and the catering of food. He seemed to interact well with others, but he was alone, lonely, and filled with self-hate. Since that meeting I have pondered his situation in life and marvelled at his personal courage to be. Somehow, not precisely in the ways that Frankl has discussed, he has risen above or transcended what could easily become a death trajectory to exhibit the courage to be.

REFERENCES

Aquinas, Thomas. 1990. "The Catholic View," in John Donnelly, ed., *Suicide: Right or Wrong?* Buffalo, N.Y.: Prometheus Books, pp. 33–36, from *Summa Theologica,* Part 2, Question 64, A5.

Eddy, James M., and Wesley F. Alles. 1983. *Death Education.* St. Louis: The C. V. Mosby Company.

Frankl, Victor E. 1963, 1969. *Man's Search for Meaning.* New York: Washington Square Press.

Hume, David. 1990. "Reason and Superstitions," in John Donnelly, ed., *Suicide: Right or Wrong?* Buffalo, N.Y.: Prometheus Books, pp. 37–45, from *The Philosophical Works of David Hume,* "On Suicide."

Larue, Gerald A. 1985. *Euthanasia and Religion.* Los Angeles: The Hemlock Society.

May, Rollo. 1975. *The Courage to Create.* New York: W. W. Norton & Company.

Wickett, Ann. 1989. *Double Exit.* Eugene, Ore.: The Hemlock Society.

19

Elder Dying, Elder Death

"Death is not the ultimate tragedy of life. The ultimate tragedy is de-personalization—dying in an alien and sterile area, separated from the spiritual nourishment that comes from being able to reach out to a loving hand, separated from a desire to experience the things that make life worth living, separated from hope."

—Norman Cousins, *Anatomy of an Illness,* p. 133

Death terminates life. As elders approach death they become aware that there are no further developmental patterns to anticipate. At other stages of human aging one may look forward to what lies ahead: a child looks forward to becoming a youth; the youth to becoming an adult; the adult anticipates marriage, career, and the establishment of the self in society. For the elder there is no developmental stage ahead. Death is the terminus.

THE FEAR OF DEATH

Does elder awareness of the approach of death produce fear? Is the coping mechanism known as "denial" the equivalent of "fear"? Victor W. Marshall (1980) summarized studies that have attempted to assess fear of death (pp. 64–78). There is no indication that old age automatically triggers fear of death. The "fear," however defined, appears across age, sex, racial, and cultural lines. Some elders fear death; others do not. Some elders (as well as those in other age brackets) can conceive of death as a "blessing"; others do not. Some fear a long process of dying in which they would become burdensome to others. In other words, assumptions about aging and fear of death must be tempered with caution.

Denial of death (when one has a terminal illness) is not necessarily a symptom of fear. It is a coping mechanism designed to distance one's self from a distasteful and upsetting reality. At some levels, denial may incorporate a form of magical thinking: "If I don't think about it, perhaps it will go away!" Denial, as Kubler-Ross (1969) recognized, provides a time buffer between the awareness of approaching death and the actual time of dying. It is a way of handling the shock of being told that an illness is terminal (pp. 34–43).

Anecdotal accounts of elders coping with death produce mixtures of humor and concern plus occasional references to specific fears. Dr. Eric Blau (1989), a physician, photographed and recorded comments from individuals who had been told by their doctors that they were terminally ill. Included in his collection are statements by:

- Ross Brown, who asked, "Who's going to screw in the lightbulb in the garage when I'm gone?" (p. 60)

- Mildred Gaulin, who said, "Who wants to hear an old lady moaning and groaning? I don't want to be a burden to anyone and that's what keeps me going. I'm just not going to give up. It's a great fear and I try not to dwell on it because I think the answer is to take each day as it comes. If things happen, they happen. That's the answer." (p. 82)

- Leroy Robbins, who summarized his life: "Fortunately, I've had what I consider to be a good life and I have more or less accomplished not only what I set out to do, but I did it as well as I could and I've had a good time doing it. I've had some rough times, but even so, I wouldn't want to have been anybody else that I know of." (p. 56)

- Wendell O'Dell, who commented, "I have lived my life the best I can. I have no fears of death. The only thing that concerns me is a lingering death that would be painful and would cause my family a lot of pain watching me." (p. 48)

- Helen Anderson who expressed her concern as follows, "My greatest fear is being a burden. My husband has been such a good husband because he takes care of me and he won't let me do things. . . . I don't want to die, but I realize that I may die. You know, we will all die." (p. 50)

Perhaps these are not the most profound statements ever uttered about life and death, and perhaps because they are anecdotal they do not summarize what people in general feel or think. No doubt, if I visited with elders living in poverty or who exist, somehow, on skid row, I would get another set of responses. Blau's reaction to these persons is that they are "common heroes" who "taught me much about living and dying" (p. 9).

Some elders fear certain aspects of death: experiencing a painful death, becoming a burden to others, dying alone and isolated. Some fear dying an undignified death, however they define the term. Perhaps the guide to understanding fear of death lies in the observation made by Robert E. Kavanaugh that "fear of death is fear of life" (1974, p. 41). Elders have lived the greatest part of their lives, and they got through it. They learned how to cope and how to manage upsetting and troublesome situations and ideas. They have no particular fear of life, because they have more or less successfully lived through most of their life. The vast majority have the courage to continue to be, despite the inconveniences that accompany terminal illnesses. It seems to me that any "fear" associated with death can be considered a natural but temporary and not paralyzing reaction to a reality. After all, although we may be at the bedside of the terminally ill and watch others die, no one knows what it is like to die until one has experienced it and then (despite the claims of those who report on near-death-experiences) it is too late to come back and report on it. Therefore, if fear of death exists, perhaps it can be linked to fear of the unknown.

COPING WITH THE END OF LIFE

There are those who argue that because the years of living are, for elders, limited, each moment must be lived as though it were a precious jewel. One should squeeze each drop of meaning and purpose from every experience so that the remaining time will encompass all that may have been omitted in the early part of the life journey. To sit, relax, read, to lie in a hammock and do nothing in particular, to participate in the ordinariness of life are exercises (or lack of exercises) to be viewed as time wasted or ill-spent because death is waiting just around the corner to cut short the potential for life-involvement.

There is some merit in resolving "to burn out rather than rust out" and in determining "to savor the bread of life to its last crumb," but even such positive responses cannot ignore the fact that life presents moments of disappointment that must be confronted, failures that must be handled, and losses that must be coped with. The proximity of death need not produce desperate responses: "run-for-your-life" or "have only positive experiences." To savor life is to taste its many flavors both positive and life-affirming as well as negative or life-denying. To seek to burn out does not ignore the reality that the routine and perhaps the monotonous are part of normality. To be pressed into desperate efforts to see all and touch all can force elders into a stressful physical and emotional marathon to hold off death, an effort that can only be health-denying.

A retired medical doctor and his wife, now in their late eighties, have determined to remain active travelers and visit as many different places as they can throughout their declining years. They sign up for cruises to far away places, enjoying the company of fellow voyagers who are their university alumni. Year by year the trips become more arduous, and their determination to keep up with the crowd drains their limited energies and the energies of cruise directors. We can admire their determination and courage even as we recognize both their fear of being locked in at home and their attempts to distance themselves from the inevitability of death. Their efforts are reminiscent of W. Somerset Maugham's short story "Appointment in Samarra," in which an individual seeks to flee death only to meet it at the place to which he has fled.

When I asked a sixty-year-old psychologist friend, "What would you do if you knew you had only two weeks to live?" he answered without hesitation, "I'd eat! I would buy an Egyptian galebeah (the long free flowing robe) and then I would eat all the things I really love but have to avoid for health reasons. I would go out stuffed!" Certainly he would not try to cram into the two weeks all the experiences in life he had missed. He would do what seemed to him to be the most desirable thing—eat! Others might make different choices. To each his (or her) own!

Like men and women who lived in earlier generations, today's elders have developed varying coping patterns to deal with death, including both their own demise and that of significant others. Some have accepted a faith system according to which they will experience rebirth or reincarnation. Other faith systems predict paradise or hell according to the way in which one has lived one's life and how one is judged by the deity or whatever court may be believed to exist in the afterlife. Obviously, this means that the Muslim paradise will feature marked differences from that anticipated by Christians, and Far Eastern reincarnation will harmonize with neither. Each system can provide help in coping with death.

Of course, there is absolutely no proof of an existence beyond death or of a paradise or a hell. Such ideas are faith statements reflecting psychological coping patterns—the denial that life really does end. The frailty of such belief systems has been commented upon in our most ancient literature (Larue 1990). What we do know is that when death does come, all awareness, all consciousness ceases and the body begins to decay.

Significant numbers of elders cope with the reality of death by taking steps to ease the impact of their demise on survivors. They write wills to make sure their intentions are carried out concerning the division of possessions. They make their own funeral arrangements to relieve others of this burden. They donate their bodies or body parts to institutions that will use them to teach through dissection or to replace defective organs in others thus enabling these others to live or live better. They make closure with persons important in their lives by expressing love and concern so that misunderstandings are eliminated and no feeling-gaps remain. They act out of an altruistic ethic that expresses love and concern for others.

Some elders may commit a posthumous suicide by destroying anything and everything that may constitute a memory of the self. It will be as if they never existed apart from official birth and death records. They withhold from the future any inheritance of their unique memories or experiences, and, at times, any expression of concern for the disposal of their possessions—indeed, almost any evidence of their being or existence. Personal records are destroyed and any property or personal items that remain are simply left for the greed of those who remain to argue over and divide.

One retired, prominent educator insisted that there be no publicity given to his death—no newspaper announcements or obituary notices and no funeral or memorial services. His body was cremated and the ashes were strewn over the ocean. Former colleagues, students, and acquaintances learned of his death by happenstance when they phoned to invite him to a luncheon or to inquire about his research or his health. And they were confused, shocked, and bewildered. What sort of anger or martyr complex or pathological rejection of others is involved in such behavior?

Some of us recall conversations with this man. He enjoyed his life, his work, his friends. He was impressed with how far humans had evolved in the 250,000 years of their existence, but was equally impressed by the awareness that it required more than six million years for them to surface after their ancestors split from the species that developed as chimpanzees and gorillas. He did not believe that evolution was divinely or otherwise directed to produce the human. We are simply one of a number of species that have adapted and survived. Moreover, because he dealt in cosmic and geological time patterns, the individual life was dwarfed to become nothing more than that, an individual life, just as a single ant is an individual ant. In other words, he did not elevate himself, glorify himself, or divinize himself. He simply was. He existed for sixty-nine years and then he was not. His concept of immortality was that life may be immortal in that it occurs in every generation but he did not accept personal immortality. He expected his friends, colleagues, and acquaintances to accept his death as they had accepted his life. Those closest to him would know of it immediately. Others would learn in time. There would be no room for public mourning, regrets, unnecessary closures, and so on. He had died. He was dead. Period. Perhaps some lives had been affected by his presence, his teaching, his writings, but that was the past and if that was to constitute his immortality, so be it.

There can be little doubt that his unannounced demise prompted reactions and some pondering. I was reminded of a poem an aunt once penned in a remembrance book:

> Remember me, 'tis all I ask,
> But if remembrance proves a task,
> Forget me.

Many of us heard of his death through phone calls from others who had learned by chance themselves. It was then that we remembered some of our conversations and it was this recall that caused us to ponder. He died as he lived, true to himself. We had to accept that. If we experienced some guilt because we "ought to have" kept in touch with him—well, that was our problem, and perhaps it would prompt us to reach out to other friends who mattered. He was not acting in a mean or cruel fashion; he was just being who he always was.

For some elders, the experience of the death of others often presents unique coping difficulties. The death of a grandchild may seem unfair: shouldn't elders die first? The closer the bonding of elder to grandchild, the greater the difficulty in accepting the basic realities of nature and of existence that sometimes shatter life patterns by disease, accident, and violence. The fact that when the elder was young, children died in large numbers from diseases that have now been largely overcome in no way eases the pain of the loss of a child today. Those earlier deaths have become distant and, moreover, as a child the elder had the support of parents. Now the elder is isolated, orphaned, even though she or he may still be part of a family unit. No one other than another elder can quite understand the unique grief an older person may experience at the death of a grandchild (see Larue 1981).

Coping with the death of an adult child may be eased intellectually by the awareness that the person lived a reasonably long life, but emotional reactions ignore the rational. The dead adult was the child raised by the elder and such a death rips away part of a history of involvement—a long history marked with transitions that gave special meaning to existence. Moreover, such a death removes a familial life support upon which the elder may no longer rely.

The most traumatic loss for married elders is that of a spouse. For unknown reasons, women seem to cope with spousal death better than men. A higher percentage of men die within a year or two following the death of a wife, than do women following the death of a husband. Perhaps because men have been taught to contain and control their emotions, their grief expressions tend to be bottled up, producing stress that contributes to death. It is likely that women have tended to form more effective support groups throughout life and these groups and the patterns of sharing feelings enable them to work through their grief in healthier ways. Then again, because men tend to live much of their lives in a business atmosphere they are far more emotionally dependent on their wives, whose adult lives have been focussed on familial interactions that have trained them to work through emotional upsets and losses.

After the death of his wife of forty-five years, a trained counselor followed all the recommended therapeutic steps for coping with loss. He participated in group sessions with other grieving elders, kept active and involved, and did not neglect physical and relaxation exercises. Nevertheless, on a given day about three months after his wife's death, the counselor found his legs had become so weak that he could not walk. He was hospitalized. No physical causes could be found for his weakness. After six weeks of rehabilitation he was able to walk again, and from that point on functioned as he always had. His explanation is simple: his weakness was a grief reaction that surfaced despite his efforts to follow the accepted guidelines for successfully coping with grief. His mind, his psyche, told him that something essential had been ripped from him, and his body responded.

Deaths of friends and colleagues remind elders of their own mortality. Some check the age of the deceased against their own age. If the person is ten years younger, he or she "died young." If the person is ten years older, that fact pushes the time of death away for at least ten years. If the person is approximately the same age, the awareness of approaching death is increased. One educator refused to attend meetings of a "sixty-five and up" group because during each meeting a list was read of ailing members and the names of those who had died. He commented, "I come to the meeting feeling fine, I leave depressed. Who needs it?"

THE PREPARATION FOR DYING AND DEATH

The preparation for dying is equal in importance to the preparation for death. Unlike the sudden or easy deaths portrayed in cinema, some elders experience a prolonged and painful death. Of course, many elders die peacefully in their sleep, while others succumb to sudden coronaries. Such deaths are swift; whatever pain is experienced is of short duration. There can be no preparation for such deaths. They just happen, without warning.

Modern medicine has engaged the skills of chemists, bioengineers, and other technicians to produce machinery that can sustain life in bodies that, at the beginning of the century, would have been dead. Kidney dialysis, respirators, and intravenous and naso-gastric feeding are supplemented by drugs that regulate breathing and/or heartbeat, that fight infections, that restore hormonal balances, and so forth. The simple pharmacy most elders remember from their childhood has been enhanced by a veritable arsenal of health-promoting and disease-fighting chemicals. In "those childhood days," doctors with their black bags of medical supplies came to the home to treat the sick, and normal medical care was the responsibility of the family. Hospitals were reserved for serious operations or to confine those suffering from contagious diseases. Today, doctors rarely if ever call upon patients in their homes; instead, patients go to the doctor's office or to the medical facility with which the doctor is associated. The little black bag has long since become passe; treatment is provided in settings where the latest and most sophisticated medical tools and facilities are immediately available.

The marvelous progress in medicine and health studies has engendered a new longevity for large numbers of people. Never before in human history have so many elders lived so long. And there is no end in sight. However, this development has produced situations and settings in which many elders experience a diminishing of control over their lives, which, in turn, produces feelings of helplessness and loss of dignity. Many years ago, when Max Ferber addressed my "Death and Dying" class, he recounted, with some anger, the tears he shed when he saw Irma, his wife, the woman he loved and with whom he had shared his life for so many years, being kept alive by medical science. She was bedridden in the hospital with tubes attached to practically every orifice of her body. Without the intubation she would have died, but her doctors viewed death as the enemy and were committed to keeping the woman alive as long as possible. For Max, her situation was the ultimate indignity, an expression of unethical medicine.

There was no law then that permitted doctors to "pull the plug" on the life-support systems they had initiated. There were no living wills. Irma was helpless and so was Max; modern medicine was in control. When she died, Max wrote that his tears were not for the loss of this beloved woman, but for the indignity she experienced in the dying process. His poignant *crie de couer* appeared in the *Los Angeles Times* in November 1975, and in the *Reader's Digest,* April 1976.

Max was not alone in his reaction. His essay provoked response. Consequently, he became an active campaigner for the 1976 California Natural Death Act, which has now been adopted in most states and in many countries. In one form or another, such acts provide that patients' wishes must be respected whether they call for having life-support systems turned off and resuscitation methods abandoned or, on the other hand, having the utmost efforts made to sustain life. To make clear just what are a patient's wishes the "Living Will" has come into being. In this document elders, and others who have reached the age for self-determination, stipulate that they are of sound mind and express their wishes concerning treatment in the event that they are involved in an accident or afflicted with a disease that produces irreversible coma or that is terminal, perhaps accompanied by intractable pain. Each person may spell out specific important personal details. In this way the tragic experience of the Ferbers will not be repeated and doctors will be permitted to abandon heroic treatment and remove life support equipment in accordance with the patient's wishes without fear of legal reprisal. Living Wills often have time limits and must be periodically updated. Each will must be properly witnessed and it is recommended that copies be distributed to next-of-kin, doctor(s), the hospital, and to one's lawyer. Such distribution will guarantee the fulfillment of the requests made in the will.

The Living Will has been supplemented by a document called "The Durable Power of Attorney for Health Care." Now elders (or any adult) may choose some person to act on their behalf should these elders be unable to make their wishes known concerning health care. The same distribution of the signed and witnessed document is recommended.

But what if an elder is terminally ill with painful bone cancer that cannot be relieved but is not on a life-support system? What if the elder is feeble, incontinent, miserable, house-bound, completely dependent upon others for the basic elements of decent survival? What choices are available?

THE HOSPICE WAY OF DYING

We don't all die peaceful deaths in our sleep at home. Some die miserable deaths marked by pain and suffering. Others die lonely deaths, isolated in hospitals or nursing homes. Still others have forewarnings of death; their physicians have given them a prognosis, a time scale, of say, six months or less, to live.

How do we cope with painful dying and with the knowledge that our remaining days are limited to six months or less? How do we handle the pain, the fears, the awareness of impending loss? Joan Craven and Florence S. Wald (1985) have specified some fundamental needs basic to coping and to meaningful dying: "What people need most when they are dying is relief from the distressing symptoms of their disease, the security of a caring environment, sustained expert care, and the assurance that their families won't be abandoned [in their grief]" (p. 1816). One response to these specific and basic needs is found in the hospice concept.

The term "hospice" is derived from the Latin word for hospitality. In the Middle Ages it described an inn or place of rest and relaxation for travelers or pilgrims. The most widely known modern hospice is St. Christopher's in London, whose founder and director is Dame Cicely Saunders, a social worker who became a medical doctor. This remarkable woman developed her hospice concept by focussing care on the needs of the patient rather than on those of the institution. Inspired by her work, hospices were opened in 1970 in the United States. Presently, there are more than 1,000 recognized hospices in operation.

Hospice was not designed specifically for the aged, therefore terminally ill persons of all ages are treated. The program provides palliative and supportive care for the dying and for their families. What is offered are carefully designed and sophisticated medical and nursing care regimens employing new pharmaceutical and other treatment methods for the control of pain, nausea, and other conditions that deprive the terminally ill of strength, the will to live, and often of human dignity. Thus hospice seeks to provide pain-free, loving, and supportive environments enabling the dying to live their remaining days as fully as possible. By acknowledging the reality of death and by recognizing that it is often accompanied by intense suffering and pain—physical, mental, and spiritual—which spills in widening circles to incorporate family, friends, caregivers, work associates, and in some instances neighbors, hospice considers the entire family to be the unit of care—care that extends into the post-death bereavement period.

Hospice provides an alternative to hospital and nursing home care for terminally ill persons who have less than six months to live. Unlike hospitals, which separate the terminally ill from other patients, hospice encourages an environment in which a variety of healthy persons are present. In other words, the intention is to make the process of dying as natural, humane, and tension free as possible. Some hospices are set in separate buildings and units, some are associated with hospitals, and others are independent of hospitals, but the bulk of hospice work is related to home care. Costs for care in hospice units approximate that of hospitals. Payments are made by the patient's family, by some (though not all) insurance companies, and by some state governments.

In home care, the family is the primary caregiver and hospice views the patient and the family as the unit of care. The hospice team provides both emotional and physical support and may include the patient's own doctor plus the hospice doctor, nurses, social workers, therapists, psychiatrists, chaplains, and volunteers. Emotional support involves empathetic listening and counseling. Physical support extends from assistance with patient care to occasional full takeover of responsibilities for a day.

Hospice recognizes three major goals. The first is to ease the physical discomfort of the patient by keeping the person as pain free and physically alert as possible. No efforts are made to effect cures and no artificial life-support systems, chemotherapy, blood tranfusions, or related life-sustaining measures are involved. Medical procedures are aimed at providing physical relief, and the only drugs and technologies employed are designed to relieve pain. In Europe, a pain-killer known as Brompton's Mixture (more familiarly "Brompton's Cocktail") was developed for the control of pain. The mixture contained Dianmorphine HCL, cocaine, alcohol (90 percent), syrup, and choloroform water. The presence of cocaine made the mixture unacceptable in the United States, inasmuch as cocaine is an addictive substance (the dying person might become addicted?) and a Hospice Mix was substituted containing morphine, alcohol, and usually one of the phenothiazines (thorazine, Pheneagen, compazine) in a water solution with cherry syrup to disguise the bitter taste. With the improvement of morphines, both Brompton's and the Hospice mixes have been modified.

Pain management is under the patient's jurisdiction and is generally self-administered by the patient on the basis of personal need. The patient keeps a personal pain chart or a "comfort chart," which provides a sense of control over his or her life and impending death. The medication keeps the patient as comfortable and alert as possible and contributes to a peaceful death, while at the same time easing family tensions induced by watching a loved one in excruciating pain.

The second goal concerns death with dignity. This aim precludes the use of rescue techniques once the patient stops breathing. What is stressed is "quality of life," which means keeping the patient alert, able to enjoy family, visitors, and surroundings; and not desensitized by pain and anxiety. In addition to visits by the patient's family, hospice workers may bring their own families, including children, to visit their patients. In some places pets are permitted, and, of course, they are not prohibited in home care. Hospice is committed to the idea that the individual as a social being can only fully manifest personhood in the presence of others, therefore the world of hospice is made up of young and old, sick and healthy, frail and strong, just as in the normal world of healthy persons.

Finally, hospice is designed to assist a patient in achieving a peaceful death. Because the term "patient" is interpreted to include the dying person's family and friends, these persons will need help in adjusting to the reality of impending death. Thus, the work of hospice begins before death and extends after death.

When the patient remains at home, hospice volunteers provide respite care, giving the family caregivers free time away from the immediate caring responsibilities and perhaps a day off, when the hospice team takes over full care for the dying person. Respite care may include reading to the patient, writing letters, feeding and bathing the patient, assistance with personal hygiene, and so forth. Thus, help is given directly to the patient and indirectly to those who will survive the death.

Hospice volunteers, who are truly the core of the program, are carefully screened and trained as members of teams. Those chosen become involved in continuing educational programs, for there is always more to learn. Volunteers choose to work in hospice programs for a variety of reasons: some out of their own experiences with hospice when a family member died, some are nurses dissatisfied with the ways hospitals deal with the dying, and others are drawn by the desire to be of service. Most selection committees try to exclude persons who may be emotionally disturbed, live in dysfunctional home settings, or who come with a religious aim to "save" the dying "before it is too late."

It should not be assumed that hospice work is simple or easy. Some patients are upset, angry, and disturbed individuals. Others are members of dysfunctional families. But disagreeable patients are not removed from the program; volunteers and team members learn to cope with such persons. Obviously, the stress involved can be more than the volunteers bargained for and therefore provisions are made for volunteers to "unload" emotional burdens. There can be no doubt that during a six-month period of close association with a dying person and the family a considerable degree of transference occurs.* The patient's death can impact on the volunteer and team members as well as on the family.

What hospice has done (and is doing) is change the environment for dying from the sterility of the hospital ward to the warmth of the family hearth (where such an environment exists). Many elders will continue to die in hospital beds, isolated from parts of their family (e.g., children and pets), sustained in life as long as possible by artificial means that cannot cure and barely keep alive. Because so few doctors and nurses are trained in the treatment of sick and dying elders, the potential for the isolation of feeble and dying elderly patients is intensified. The high cost of medical care may indirectly help to encourage home treatment, but assistance to ease the strain on a burdened and busy family may not be readily available, thus tending to increase tensions and pave the way for neglect and abuse of terminally ill elders. In such circumstances, the hospice program becomes truly beneficial.

The hospice way of dying is affecting the treatment of elders in hospitals, in nursing homes, and in families. The focus changes and begins to center on the value and meaning of the lived life rather than on the length of life; and on the dignity and inestimable value or sacredness of the person. Death is accepted as the normal, natural termination of life, and every effort is made to maintain respect and dignity for that life up to the very last breath.

The ethical concerns that govern hospice are, or should be, as follows:

1. *A recognition that persons die in different ways and that each person should have the right to choose his or her manner of dying.* Each disease impacts in its own way and therefore the unique requirements of each patient must be recognized. Although the majority of patients in a hospice

---

*"Transference" refers to emotions directed toward the volunteer. In the mind of the patient the caseworker's status becomes less that of a visiting professional and more that of a very special family member.

program tend to be cancer victims, the aim is to make the dying process, no matter what the disease, as comfortable as possible for the patient and the family. What is most important for elders is that the health field is focused on the importance of the personhood of the dying patient.

2. Hospice allows dying elders to be involved in their own demise by recognizing that *patients should have the right to participate in all decisions concerning treatment,* including such ordinary matters as choice of foods, beverages, and so forth. Insofar as possible, hospice puts dying elders in control of their own pain medication, which helps patients to remain alert and dignifies elders' rights to choose at what moment medication is to be taken.

3. Dying elders are to be *treated with honesty,* and if questions asked cannot be answered then the patient will be so informed without efforts to divert the question or stall as a result of ignorance. Forthright answers combat feelings of fear and uncertainty.

4. Dying elders *will not be ignored or abandoned, but will receive care, comfort, and understanding.* Wherever possible, family and friends, visitors, and even pets are integrated into the caregiving process.

5. *Dying elders will know that after death the family will be supported with care and understanding.* This awareness removes a source of worry for older adults who may have vivid recollections of the feelings of being orphaned when their parents died.

Concerns for human and personal dignity underly the hospice concept, which represents a geroethical statement and expression of the highest order. It provides an ethical response to the elder patient's need for autonomy, control, and dignity in dying.

EUTHANASIA

What if the elder does not want to continue living? Is it possible that in the lifetime of an elder, a day may come when the innate survival instinct is rendered null and void and a greater ethical principle, namely, the right to choose to die, takes precedent? The answer must be yes. It is that moment when the quality of the individual's personal life has decayed; when the meaning of life, no matter how defined, has eroded; when relationships may still be important but secondary to the need to escape from living; when existence, even in a hospice setting, has become burdensome and death is to be preferred over life—in such a moment the individual's right to choose death must be acknowledged as an ethical choice.

Who chooses that moment? The dying person does. No one can define quality of life for another. Obviously, there is some risk in acknowledging freedom to choose death. Almost any suicide might be attributed to loss of meaning in life. Many suicides result from impulsive, disorderly, and irrational thinking. For the moment, the individual is convinced that life is not worth living, but if the disturbed and troubled person can be dissuaded, at least temporarily, from self-killing, then, in the light of a new day, besetting problems can assume different dimensions and solutions to what appeared to be insurmountable barriers can be found.

But there is another level of self-killing that reflects rational evaluation of a present setting and a reasonable prognosis of what lies ahead. If for example, the medical analysis reveals that the patient is in pain and terminally ill with only a few months or weeks to live; that all medical treatments have been exhausted; that the future gives promise of continuing pain, fatigue, and frustration; then choosing to die can be recognized as a rational and perhaps an acceptable alternative to continuing to live. And if that elder wants to die, what can be done in such a situation? One answer is euthanasia.

Euthanasia, from the Greek *eu,* meaning "good," and *thanatos,* meaning "death," conveys the concept of a beneficent death or, perhaps, an acceptable death. In our present time, euthanasia is linked to the concern for dying with dignity.

Euthanasia may be voluntary or involuntary, passive or active. Voluntary euthanasia refers to the causing of death at the request of the individual; involuntary euthanasia signifies that the patient has not given consent. Passive euthanasia refers to the abandonment of heroic means of preserving life in terminally ill patients, perhaps by foregoing or withdrawing life-support systems. Voluntary passive euthanasia occurs in accordance with the patient's wishes or request, as expressed in a living will or through someone designated to have the durable power of attorney for health care. Most hospitals and most doctors honor the patient's request; some few still refuse to comply. The removal of life-support equipment without the patient's approval would constitute involuntary passive euthanasia and would be unethical, even if well meant. Passive euthanasia is sometimes referred to as "letting die."

Active euthanasia signifies that someone acts to cause the patient's death by providing lethal medication or by involvement in any death-inducing act. Voluntary active euthanasia refers to causing death at the patient's request: involuntary active euthanasia would be causing death without the patient's consent and would automatically be unethical. In either case, the act is generally treated as homicide and is against the law.

Where patients are able, they may take their own lives by committing suicide, as did Bruno Bettelheim who swallowed sedatives then pulled a plastic bag over his head, secured it by a rubber band at the neck, and died quietly in his sleep from suffocation. Others have used barbiturates (Humphry 1984). If another person gives assistance, by providing the means of suicide (e.g., providing the sedatives or attaching the plastic bag) that person can be prosecuted on the basis of assisting or abetting a suicide.

Presently there is a movement to legalize a form of active euthanasia known as "physician aid-in-dying" (Risley 1987). Groups of concerned persons, including many elders, seek to have enacted laws aimed at providing "a humane and dignified death" by which a caring physician, in response to the request of a suffering, terminally ill patient, would, without fear of prosecution, provide lethal medication to cause death. On November 5, 1991, citizens in the State of Washington were given the opportunity to vote for Initiative 119, which would have established physician assistance in dying for the terminally ill. Aggressive television campaigns were launched by those opposing the initiative (most often right-to-life groups) and by those supporting it. It was defeated by a 53.6 percent to 46.4 percent vote. Analysis of the failure of the initiative to carry (according to polls, it had a substantial margin for success) suggested that it failed to provide adequate safeguards to protect against involuntary deaths of patients who were elderly, poor, or otherwise vulnerable. Nevertheless, the 46.4 percent vote has been interpreted by some as an indication of the public's lack of confidence in medicine's ability to control pain in terminal illness.

On December 1, 1991, a new law went into effect called the Patient Self-Determination Act. It is the first federal act to address end-of-life decision making. The law requires that all federally funded health-care institutions such as Health Maintenance Organizations (HMOs), hospitals, home health agencies, skilled nursing facilities, hospice programs, and Medicare and Medicaid programs *must* inform patients of their right to prepare advance directives for their care in these institutions, and to have their documented wishes carried out. Before or at admission, patients must be informed in writing of their right to accept or refuse particular medical treatment while they are competent to make decisions, and about the care to be received should competence be lost. Handouts must be presented detailing exactly what the particular state statutes or case law permits as well as the institution's policy as it affects patient rights. New patients must be asked if a Living Will or Durable Power of Attorney for Health Care has been prepared. If such exists, the document should become a permanent part of the patient's medical record.

A Humane and Dignified Death Act has been proposed for California. At the time of writing, enough signatures have been gathered to place the measure on the ballot. It, too, seeks to legalize physician aid in dying, but this proposal contains the important safeguards missing in the Washington Initiative. Plans are underway for similar efforts in other states.

Holland has been a torchbearer in physician assisted euthanasia. Although euthanasia remains on the penal code as a violation of law, if certain criteria are followed, the courts will "excuse" the act (Admiraal 1986). The criteria are as follows:

- the patient must be competent (which would exclude patients in advance stages of Alzheimer's disease or those in a persistent vegetative state);

- the act is voluntary;

- the request for aid in dying is enduring, consistent, well-documented, and made repeatedly (as opposed to being a sudden impulse);

- the patient experiences intolerable mental and/or physical suffering, which is to say the patient need not be terminal (depression alone would not be an acceptable reason);

- the physician has tried all alternatives acceptable to the patient to relieve the suffering;

- both patient and doctor acknowledge the cognitive deterioration that can come with end-stages of the illness; and

- euthanasia must be performed by the attending doctor in consultation with another physician not involved in the case.

The procedure may involve the ingesting of a barbiturate (to induce sleep) mixed with powdered orphenadrine* combined with yogurt and sugar to

---

*Orphenadrine is combined pharmaceutically with less toxic drugs in prescription for the treatment of some forms of Parkinson's Disease. In Holland, the lethal three-gram dosage of the unadulterated drug is used to produce death.

mask the bitter taste. The patient dies within twenty minutes (Admiraal, "Euthanasia," 1988). On other occasions the barbiturate is followed by a lethal injection or curare* (Angell 1988). Although euthanasia often takes place in nursing homes and hospital settings, it is commonly performed in homes, where the patient can be with members of the family.

In these latter settings, there is, in a sense, a return to pre-institutionalizing patterns of patient care to provide a setting that many consider to be more humane, more comfortable, and more compassionate than death in a hospital. In each case, the doctor acts in response to the request of the patient. The patient is provided with the opportunity to make final farewells and, at an agreed upon time, perhaps in the presence of immediate family members, both young and old, the doctor administers a lethal injection that brings on a painless and rapid death. As in times past, the patient dies with the family close by. Now, instead of "letting nature take its course," which could involve a lengthy period of pain and suffering, the patient dies quietly and easily, knowing that she or he has been in charge of living and dying up to the last breath. There is dignity in such dying. There is dignity in such a death.

Naturally, active euthanasia is not for everyone. In the United States and in other countries, active voluntary euthanasia and doctor-assisted death are forbidden by law. In other words, should a terminally ill person in intractable pain request help in dying from his or her doctor, that request would, out of fear of prosecution alone, probably be refused or ignored. Numerous medical practitioners have admitted that they have, at the request of a terminally ill patient, administered medications that brought on death. Some have argued that overdoses of morphine are given to control pain even in the full awareness that the overdose will cause death. These megadoses, the argument goes, are to be classified as efforts in pain-control, not as euthanasia. The language is, of course, protective to avoid criminal prosecution; nevertheless, the act is euthanasia no matter how physicians seek to mask it.

Surveys have indicated that eight out of ten Americans think there are circumstances in which a patient should be permitted to die, heroic means of sustaining life should be abandoned, and life-support systems should be removed according to the patient's wishes. In such instances

---

*Curare is a resinlike substance obtained from plants of the *Strychnos* genus or from the root of the South American vine called pareira. South American Indians once used it to poison their arrows. In modern medicine, curare is employed in combination with other substances as a relaxant. Used in its pure form in an injection, it is lethal.

the Living Will and Durable Power of Attorney for Health Care, properly executed and witnessed, become powerful implements. Millions of copies of both documents have been distributed, filled out, witnessed, and shared with family members, doctors, lawyers, and hospitals. Such sharing provides the physician and the hospital opportunity to express their willingness or unwillingness to comply with the patient's expressed wishes. Where non-compliance is indicated, the patient can look for another doctor and/or hospital. The Living Will has been given legal status in some thirty-seven states and the Durable Power of Attorney for Health Care is receiving growing acceptance.

These documents do not always serve to protect the person. In emergency situations following a heart attack or serious injury, paramedics may be initially in charge of the victim as the patient is rushed to a hospital emergency room. In such traumatic settings the documents have little relevance since, in emergency cases there is an implied assumption of patient consent. Emergency health professionals are trained to rescue and save life, and once procedures have been initiated they can be very hard to stop.

Where such documents have not been signed, the situation can become complicated. For example, when Nancy Cruzan, a thirty-two-year-old victim of an automobile accident was in a vegetative state for seven years and was kept alive by a feeding tube, requests made by her parents to remove the feeding tube were refused by the Supreme Court because there was no solid evidence that such an act would be in accord with her wishes. She had not signed a Living Will, and like many young people, had given little thought to dying. It was only after some former friends became aware of her situation and testified to the fact that she had, in their presence, declared that she would not want to be kept alive under such circumstances that the courts permitted the removal of the life-sustaining feeding tube so that Ms. Cruzan could die. There are those who would argue that the Cruzan case was a far more acceptable case for intrusive active euthanasia than the Janet Adkins case, which was previously discussed. Many AIDS patients have made euthanasia plans as they experience the worsening of their conditions. The number of elders preferring to seek termination of life in similar situations is on the increase.

The issue of euthanasia can be argued on theoretical or on a case-by-case basis. It is when such cases become personal that the real ethical criteria surface. Just suppose that you, the reader, were diagnosed as having Alzheimer's Disease. You have seen what this terrible ailment does to humans because you happen to know a woman who has degenerated into childlike dependency on her husband. He talks to her in the language of a child and in tones of a condescending parent. He takes her to the toilet where she cannot care for herself. He bathes her and watches over her as if she were an infant. He listens to her comments that seem to come out of nowhere and responds kindly as if they had meaning or substance. The woman is healthy and may live another ten or fifteen years. As each year passes, she slips a little further away from reality into the fog of her brain-damaged netherworld. This is what lies ahead for you. What is your choice: to continue to live knowing that you will ultimately exist in this totally dependent fashion, or to take steps to forestall such an existence?

This is what confronted Jane Elaine Adkins, a fifty-four-year-old Oregon woman, to whom reference has been made in the discussion of dementing illness (chapter 15). She had always been a vital, involved person with a zest for life that led her to climb mountains, experiment with gliders and hot-air balloons, teach in a community college, and help immigrants and refugees to become self-sufficient. She was also a very determined person, and when she began to experience the onset of what was diagnosed as Alzheimer's Disease, she decided that she did not want to live with increasing memory loss and ultimate dementia. She sought the assistance of Dr. Jack Kevorkian, a Detroit pathologist, who had invented a machine that would enable a person who was hooked up to it to press a button and release a lethal dosage into the body thereby inducing coma and then heart failure. Janet Adkins and her husband flew to Detroit where she was carefully interviewed and evaluated by Dr. Kevorkian and other experts. On June 3, 1990, while her husband and a close family friend waited in a nearby hotel, she sat in Kevorkian's camper in a parking lot, 2,300 miles from her Portland home, and pressed the button that triggered the infusion of lethal drugs. She was in charge. She decided how and when she was to die. Was her choice ethical or unethical?

It has been argued that Janet Adkins might have waited a while longer before taking her own life. After all, she was not terminally ill and it was clear that there was still time for many good moments to be shared with friends and family. On the other hand, it must be recognized that there is no way of determining the pace of Alzheimer's Disease. Janet Adkins chose not to take chances with her future. She did not act in haste. She had tried experimental treatment. She had talked with her minister and engaged in family counseling with her sons. Then she made her decision. What is regrettable is that she was compelled to travel so far for help in dying and that she could not be in her home with her family during her final moments of life. There are those who would like to see changes made to accommodate persons like Janet Adkins in their wish to die with dignity.

Dr. Kevorkian, despite his well-meant intentions to be of help, has come under considerable criticism. He cannot be a model for carefully legislated right-to-die programs. Inasmuch as he acted as an individual, without proper safeguards for the protection of patient rights, he has been assessed as a handicap to the development of legislation designed to promote patients' rights to choose death. Nevertheless, he has dramatically brought to the attention of the American public the desperate needs of persons like Janet Adkins and the other two women whom he helped to die.

Derek Humphry, who assisted Jean, his first wife, to terminate her suffering when they lived in England, has founded The National Hemlock Society, which supports active euthanasia for the terminally ill. Humphry has recounted the story of the beginning of this important movement in the last pages of his book *Jean's Way*. I became the first president of Hemlock because I was convinced of the reasonableness and the moral justice of the arguments supporting active voluntary euthanasia for the terminally ill. Of course, not everyone agrees with this idea and strong opposition comes from those whose ethical commitment is derived from a particular interpretation of the idea of the "sanctity of life" (an idea that I support but interpret differently) or through fear of what has been called "the slippery slope."

The so-called slippery slope argument suggests that while active euthanasia may be initially directed toward the needs of the terminally ill, it is just possible that the boundaries could be expanded to include other groups. The most often quoted example supporting such fears refers to the extermination policies employed by the Nazis in World War II in which the groups designated for death in the gas chambers became more and more inclusive.

In response, Hemlock stresses the importance of rule by law, the need to enact protective euthanasia legislation, and points out that we are not Nazis. There can be no question that laws can be violated but such violations must be prosecuted to the fullest extent of the law. Until laws governing medically induced active euthanasia come into being, individuals and couples will continue to commit what Humphry has called "the compassionate crime," which is when one acts secretly, in compliance with a terminally ill person's request, to terminate pain, suffering, and misery. Some of these "compassionate crimes" committed by elders have been discovered and prosecuted as homicides with penalties ranging from probation to incarceration. The burden of responsibility for taking the life of a loved one is always heavy and although there is sorrow over the loss of a spouse, there appears to be little or no residue of guilt for having terminated a life. The act can be interpreted as a supreme expression of love and caring.

Some couples are so closely bonded that they cannot conceive of life without each other. When they become old and feeble, they make a death pact and agree to die simultaneously. Some ingest barbiturates that they have stockpiled. At times, one partner kills the other and then commits suicide, thus combining active involuntary euthanasia (murder) with suicide. Sometimes the act is successful, sometimes only one dies and the other survives.

In 1975, Dr. Henry Pitney Van Dusen, former president of Union Theological Seminary, New York, and his wife committed double suicide. He had suffered a stroke and she was crippled with arthritis. As prominent Christian educators, they were familiar with the social and religious taboos associated with self-killing, but they felt that they had been kept alive by modern medicine beyond the time they would normally have died. Their act of self-destruction is only one of an increasing number of double suicides. Ann Wickett has estimated that the rate of double suicides has increased tenfold in the period between 1980 and 1987 over what it was in the previous sixty-year period between 1920 and 1980 (Wickett 1989, p. 131). She found that in about one-half of the cases, both husband and wife suffered from a terminal illness; in about one-third of the cases, only the wife was terminal, in 19 percent only the husband was terminal (ibid., p. 141). Once again, the numbers suggest that the male elder has greater difficulty in coping with the potential loss of a spouse than the female. Meaningful longevity is clearly related to health factors (see chapter 11). In some cases, death appears to be preferable to life.

What are the ethical issues involved? The first has to do with freedom of choice—the right to choose the manner and time of one's death. There is no law against suicide per se, but if the intention to commit suicide is made known, preventive steps will be taken and the person may be confined for psychological observation. Ultimately, when individual elders choose to take their own lives, or when an elderly couple decides to die together, moral judgment becomes the problem of the survivors, not of the victims. In most cases of elder suicide, condemnations are few and there is a general understanding of the reasons behind the act. Most religious organizations respond to the deaths with compassion and without condemnation.

An ethical issue related to medically assisted euthanasia involves doctor-patient relationships. Has any patient the right to ask a doctor to give an injection that causes death? Does not such an act make the doctor a murderer? Does the request invite the doctor to turn away from his deepest desires and professional intentions to effect cures and stave off death (Maguire 1975)? Would participation in active euthanasia invite fear of doctors by a public that prefers to think of doctors as those who protect and preserve life rather than those who take it?

Some doctors have endorsed the concerns expressed above. Others have said that, for personal or religious reasons, they would not participate in active euthanasia. Many doctors have admitted that they have taken action that has brought on the death of a patient. As discussed above, some have given megadoses of morphine as pain treatment, knowing full well that the dosage would cause death. Their act was one of compassion and performed in response to the urgent pleas of a suffering patient. Nevertheless, under present law they could, if identified, be prosecuted for murder.

In November 1987, the National Hemlock Society conducted a survey among 5,000 medical doctors in the State of California. They received a 12 percent response (588). In that sample, 80 percent said that they regularly treated terminally ill patients. Almost 95 percent of those who admitted being asked to hasten death acknowledged that the request was, in their opinion, "rational." Sixty-two percent indicated that they believed it was sometimes right to agree to hasten a patient's death, and nearly 23 percent admitted that they had already helped patients to die (The National Hemlock Society 1988). A database of 676 doctors surveyed by the San Francisco Medical Society in 1988 indicated that 54 percent favored euthanasia and 45 percent said they would participate in euthanasia (Krieger 1988). It seems apparent that physician-assisted death has considerable support within the medical community and that the fears or concerns expressed above are not those of the majority of physicians who responded to the surveys.

There is considerable public support for physician-assisted suicide. In a 1986 Roper poll of 2,000 Americans, 62 percent supported physician induced euthanasia (Roper 1986), and a poll of 501 persons in Florida in 1987 indicated that 58 percent supported the idea (Humphry 1987). As noted above, the issue will soon be put to a vote in California and later in other states.

Perhaps public interest in this subject can be measured, in part, by the response to the book *Final Exit,* by Derek Humphry. The book, which provides information about "the practicalities of self-deliverance and assisted suicide for the dying" was on the bestseller list for fifteen weeks, has sold more than a half-million copies and is being translated into eight languages. It is banned in Australia and New Zealand! Until legislation is passed legalizing physician-assisted euthanasia, this book may prove to be the best friend of the terminally ill who wish to end their lives.

Meanwhile, some medical doctors will continue to act out of compassion and provide the means, or personally act, to terminate the life of a terminally ill, suffering patient. Some years ago, I received a phone call from a university professor in Canada. Her mother was dying of cancer and was in agony that could only be partially controlled by palliatives, which left her groggy and semi-comatose. She begged her daughter to do something to bring on her death. The professor asked, "What can I do?" How could I advise someone whom I had never met and who lived several thousand miles away? I said, "Talk to your doctor."

Several troublesome days passed and then I phoned the hospital room (I had noted all the necessary telephone numbers). The professor answered. "I am so glad you phoned," she said. "I have just given my mother the lethal injection. She is completely relaxed, her breathing is getting shallower and she has that wonderful little smile on her face."

She related what had taken place. After I had talked with her, she spoke to her doctor. "This morning he came down the hall and put a syringe in my hand and said that he never wanted to talk with me about this again." The professor had had time to talk with her mother, to achieve a warm and loving closure, and to assure her mother that she was ready to fulfill her mother's often repeated request to die, to be released from pain.

About fifteen months later the professor was in California attending a conference, and we finally had the opportunity to meet. She was radiant. She had expressed her love in a positive and caring way, and she had shortened the time of her mother's suffering. She had no regrets, no guilt, only peace and joy in the knowledge that this death-producing act was a statement of love.

Was the doctor's provision of the syringe and the lethal drug unethical? Was the daughter's act immoral? Legally, she had committed murder and the doctor had aided and abetted that murder. They had both violated the law. If the doctor's act had become known, there would have been those who would seek to revoke his license to practice medicine on grounds of unethical conduct. Is the label "a compassionate crime" enough to excuse their behavior?

A further question is raised by active euthanasia. Does not active voluntary euthanasia ignore or deny belief in the sanctity of human life? One response to the question can be given in the form of another question. Which act testifies to a belief in the sanctity of life—to stand by and do nothing when a terminally ill person in intractable pain begs for aid in dying, or to act in response to the person's suffering and administer a lethal medication that causes death? Does one express belief in the sanctity of life by letting a terminally ill person linger on in pain against that person's wishes? Or does one express belief in the sanctity of life by refusing to let the last hours of a precious life be marred by suffering? Each individual must decide on the basis of his or her own ethical stance.

Among the fears of the consequences of legalizing physician-assisted suicide is the suggestion that "the right to die may become a duty to die" (Capron 1987, p. 51). It is true that because the United States health-care costs can place tremendous financial burdens on families, some elders may not wish their prolonged illness to become burdensome for their families. Perhaps such elders might be persuaded that when they become frail, feeble, and ill, they have a duty to die and so ease the family financial burdens. Perhaps such responses will not be relevant when a national health insurance program comes into being, but there are those who feel that nursing and hospital costs for the dying rob the next generation. Such complaints are not new; they occur with each generation, but each generation seems to be able to manage despite such fears. What such arguments may prey upon is the inherited ethic of the nobility of self-sacrifice, which calls for the individual to place the welfare of the group above that of self. Examples usually include stories of parents sacrificing themselves for their children (or vice versa) or of the soldier who hurls himself on the grenade to protect his comrades. For Christians, the supreme example of unselfish heroic action is found in Jesus who, according to Christian theology, died for the sins of others. The presence of such thinking could place unfair burdens on elders who could be made to feel that, inasmuch as they are no longer useful or contributing members of society, they should become useful by getting out of the way and not become burdens to either family or the public. In other words, they should sacrifice themselves for the greater good.

Other fears have been expressed. Some have suggested that the legalization of active euthanasia, despite protective laws, could lead to abuse. Greedy relatives may be willing to hasten or encourage, through subtle coercion, the death of a long-lingering elder thereby maximizing the amount of money to be inherited. Furthermore, doctors have been known to make mistakes; therefore, a person diagnosed as terminal and put to death might have recovered, given enough time. In response, one must have little faith in our legal system and in our medical profession to endorse such thinking. It is true that unethical relatives are known to exist. It is also true that mistakes have been made in both the law and medicine—the law has been subverted and doctors have erred in diagnoses. But is it ethical to deny medically assisted active euthanasia to terminally ill persons who have signed the proper documents and who have worked through their decision with their doctor and with others, perhaps including their clergy and a hospital ethics committee, simply because of the fear that the choice might not be freely made, or out of fear that the doctor may have misdiagnosed the illness (Khuse, "The Alleged Peril . . ." 1987, pp. 62ff)? Doctors have been trained to recognize terminal illnesses. Moreover, a diagnosis that a disease is terminal should be based on more than a single doctor's analysis, particularly if active euthanasia is contemplated. Perhaps there have been and will be ruthless physicians who feel compelled to get rid of older patients for one reason or another. If such doctors exist, they can be recognized and their actions controlled by regulations.

In the event that medically induced voluntary active euthanasia is legalized, it is doubtful that elders will rush to die. Some persons, both young and old, have declared their intention to take their own lives as the pain associated with their terminal illnesses moves out of their control. Perhaps some of these people will seek medical help when that time comes. The cases appear to be relatively few. Not every ailing elder will choose euthanasia. Far more important is the freedom to choose. The knowledge that medical aid in dying is available will provide the terminally ill with the comfort of being assured of a dignified death at the time of their own choosing.

Finally, and what is most important, is the recognition of the right of any physician or institution to refuse to be associated in any way with active euthanasia. Not every doctor is willing to be involved in taking the life of a patient. Personal religious, professional and philosophical beliefs may forbid participation. There will also be hospitals, hospices, and other caregiving institutions that will refuse to perform active euthanasia. These are legitimate moral and ethical stands that must be respected. It is up to the patient and the patient's family to make clear their personal wishes, and if the doctor or institution are not in agreement, then another physician or institution must be found. Both the doctor and the institution have the ethical responsibility to make known to the patient their position on this very controversial issue.

REFERENCES

Admiraal, Pieter V. 1986. "Euthanasia Applied at a General Hospital," *The Euthanasia Review* 1, no. 2, pp. 97–107.
———. 1988. "Euthanasia in the Netherlands," *The Euthanasia Review* 3, no. 2, pp. 79–86.
———. 1988. "Drug Combinations are Superior," *Hemlock Quarterly,* no. 31 (April), p. 3.
Angell, Marcia. 1988. "Euthanasia," *The New England Journal of Medicine* 319, no. 20 (November 17).
Baird, Robert M., and Stuart E. Rosenbaum, eds. 1989. *Euthanasia: The Moral Issues.* Buffalo: N.Y.: Prometheus Books.
Bender, David L., and Bruno Leone, eds. 1989. *Euthanasia: Opposing Viewpoints.* San Diego, Calif.: Greenhaven Press.
Blau, Eric. 1989. *Common Heroes: Facing a Life Threatening Illness.* Pasadena, Calif.: New Sage Press.
Capron, Alexander Morgan. 1987. "The Right to Die: Progress and Peril," *The Euthanasia Review* 2, no. 2, pp. 41–59.
Chase, Deborah. 1986. *Dying at Home with Hospice.* St. Louis, Mo.: C. V. Mosby Co.
Cohen, Kenneth P. 1979. *Hospice Prescription for Terminal Care.* Germantown, Md.: Aspen Systems Corporation.
Corr, Charles A., and Donna M. Corr, eds. 1983. *Hospice Care: Principles and Practice.* New York: Springer Publishing Co.
Craven, Joan, and Florence S. Wald. 1985. "Hospice Care for Dying Patients," *The American Journal of Nursing* 75, no. 10 (October), pp. 1816–22.
Davidson, Glen. 1978. *The Hospice: Development and Administration.* New York: Hemisphere Publishing Corp.
Davidson, G. W. 1979. "Five Models for Hospice Care," *Quality Review Bulletin* 5, no. 5 (May), pp. 8–9.
DuBois, Paul M. 1980. *The Hospice Way of Death.* New York: Human Sciences Press.
Evans, M., et al. 1981. "Expect the Unexpected When You Care for a Dying Patient," *Nursing* (December), pp. 55–56.
Ferber, Max. 1975, 1976. "I Cried, Not for Irma, but for the Ignominious Way of Her Going," *The Los Angeles Times,* November 26; *The Reader's Digest,* April.
Fletcher, Joseph. 1987–88. "The Courts and Euthanasia," *Law, Medicine and Health Care* 15, no. 4 (Winter), pp. 223–30.

Gelman, David, and Karen Springen. n.d. "The Doctor's Suicide Van," *Newsweek.*

Hamilton, Michael, and Helen Reid. 1980. *A Hospice Handbook, A New Way to Care for the Dying.* Grand Rapids, Mich.: Wm. B. Eerdmans.

Hay, Jean. 1985. "An Experience in Listening," *The American Journal of Hospice Care* (May/June), pp. 45–46.

Holden, C. 1976. "Hospices: For the Dying, Relief from Pain and Fear," *Science,* no. 193, pp. 389–91.

Humphry, Derek. 1978. *Jean's Way.* New York: Harper & Row. (Reprint with supplement, 1986.)

———. 1984. *Let Me Die Before I Wake.* Eugene, Ore.: The Hemlock Society.

———. 1987. "Roper Poll Shows Support for Euthanasia," *The Euthanasia Review* 2, nos. 1–2, pp. 76–79.

———. 1991. *Final Exit.* Eugene, Ore.: The Hemlock Society.

Jacobsen, Gary A. 1979. "Hospice: A Concept of Terminal Care," *Portland Physician* (July), pp. 1–5.

Jeffers, Frances C., and Ariaan Verwoerdt. 1969. "How the Old Face Death," in Ewald Busse and Eric Pfeiffer, eds., *Behavior and Adaptions in Late Life.* Boston: Little, Brown and Company, pp. 163–81.

Jenkins, Lowell, and Alicia S. Cook. 1981. "The Rural Hospice: Integrating Formal and Informal Helping Systems," *Social Work* (September), pp. 414–16.

Kavanaugh, Robert E. 1974. *Facing Death.* New York: Penguin Books.

Kevorkian, Jack. 1991. *Prescription Medicide: The Goodness of Planned Death.* Buffalo, N.Y.: Prometheus Books.

Khuse, Helga. 1987. *The Sanctity-of-Life Doctrine in Medicine: A Critique.* Oxford: Clarendon Press.

———. 1987. "The Alleged Peril of Active Voluntary Euthanasia: A Reply to Alexander Morgan Capron," *The Euthanasia Review* 2, no. 1–2, pp. 76–79.

Koff, T. H. 1980. *Hospice: A Caring Community.* Cambridge, Mass.: Winthrop Publishers.

Kohl, Marvin. 1975. *Beneficent Euthanasia.* Buffalo, N.Y.: Prometheus Books.

Kohn, J. 1976. "Hospice Movement Provides Human Alternative for Terminally Ill Patients," *Modern Health Care,* pp. 25–29.

Kohut, Jeraldine J. 1984. *Hospice: Caring for the Terminally Ill.* Springfield, Ill.: Charles C. Thomas.

Krieger, Lisa M. 1988. "S.F. Doctors' Survey Shows 54 Percent Favor Euthanasia," *San Francisco Examiner* (May 17).

Kubler-Ross, Elisabeth. 1969. *On Death and Dying.* New York: The Macmillan Company.

Kutscher, Austin H., et al., eds. 1983. *Hospice U.S.A.* New York: Columbia University Press.

Larue, Gerald A. 1981. "The Death of a Child," *The Humanist* 41, no. 1, pp. 32, 36, 66.

———. 1985. *Euthanasia and Religion.* Los Angeles: The Hemlock Society.

Little, Deborah Whiting. 1985. *Home Care for the Dying.* Garden City, N.Y.: The Dial Press, Doubleday & Co.

Marshall, Victor W. 1980. *Last Chapters: A Sociology of Aging and Dying.* Monterey, Calif.: Brooks/Cole Publishing Co.

McCabe, S. V. 1982. "An Overview of Hospice Care," *Cancer Nursing* 2, no. 5 (April), pp. 103–107.

McDonnell, Alice. 1986. *Quality Hospice Care: Administration, Organization and Models.* Owing Mills, Md.: National Health Publication.

McNulty, Elizabeth G., and Robert A. Holderby. 1983. *Hospice: A Caring Challenge.* Springfield, Ill.: Charles C. Thomas.

Mor, Vincent. 1987. "Hospice," *Generations* (Spring), pp. 19–21.

Munley, Anne. 1983. *The Hospice Alternative: A New Context for Death and Dying.* New York: Basic Books.

Parachini, Allan. 1984. "Hospice Rated Only on a Par with Hospitals," *The Los Angeles Times,* May 1.

Paradis, Lenora Finn, ed. 1985. *Hospice Handbook: A Guide for Managers and Planners.* Rockville, Md.: Aspen Systems Corporation

Parkes, C. Murray. 1985. "The Dying Patient: Terminal Care: Home, Hospital or Hospice?" *The Lancet* (January 19), p. 155–57.

Ramsey, Paul. 1975. *The Ethics of Fetal Research.* New Haven, Conn.: Yale University Press.

Risley, Robert L. 1986. "What the Humane and Dignified Death Initiative Does," *The Euthanasia Review* 1, no. 4, pp. 221–25.

———. 1987. *A Humane and Dignified Death Act.* Glendale, Calif.: Americans Against Human Suffering.

Roper Poll. 1986. "Public Attitudes on the Legalization of Euthanasia," *The Euthanasia Review* 1, no. 3, pp. 177–75.

Saunders, Dame Cicely. 1977. "Dying They Live: St. Christopher's Hospice," in Herman Feifel, ed., *New Meanings of Death.* New York: McGraw-Hill Book Company, pp. 153–79.

———. 1988. "The Evolution of the Hospices," in R. D. Mann, ed., *The History and Management of Pain.* N.J.: The Parthenon Publishing Group, Inc., pp. 167–78.

Stoddard, Sandol. 1978. *The Hospice Movement: A Better Way of Caring for the Dying.* New York: Stein and Day.

Taylor, Jean. 1987. "Hospice House: A Homelike Inpatient Unit," *Generations,* pp. 22–26.

The National Hemlock Society. 1988. "November 1987 Survey of California Physicians Regarding Voluntary Active Euthanasia for the Terminally Ill," *The National Hemlock Society,* Eugene, Ore.

Wald, Florence S., Zelda Foster, and Henry J. Wald. 1960. "The Hospice Movement as a Health Care Reform," *Nursing Outlook* (March), pp. 173–78.

Wickett, Ann. 1989. *Double Exit.* Eugene, Ore.: The Hemlock Society.

Zimmerman, Jack M. 1986. *Hospice: Complete Care for the Terminally Ill.* Baltimore: Urban and Swarzenberg.

20

Geroethics and the Future

"The direction of the trend of cultural changes in our attitudes toward aging is toward a clearer recognition of the great riches which the aging have to contribute to our society and the betterment of mankind."

—Ashley Montagu, "The Problems of an Aging Population," 1960

Basic to the discussion of geroethics are themes such as honor, truth, love, respect, autonomy, freedom, duty, concern for the self, and concern for others. Throughout this book, social awareness of the dramatic population shifts that have occurred and are occurring in First World countries has been expressed. We estimate that by the year 2030, one-in-five Americans, 20 percent of the people, will be over sixty-five years of age. This means that students who are in my classes today will be moving into the role of elder. Five percent of the population, or one-in-twenty will then be eighty-five years of age or older and there will be several hundred thousand centenarians.

We can surmise that some, if not most, of those in the Western world who will be over sixty-five years of age will continue to be employed; some will not. It is important that the young men and women who will compose this growing elder population give thought today to preparing for the time when they will become elders. The involvement of today's youth and those who are middle-aged in bettering the health and well-being of today's elders will have significant implications for the time when they become elders.

Everything today's elders do now can influence patterns of aging in the future. Can the future learn from us? Can today's elders contribute to the brave new world that is even now beginning to emerge? What can we suggest to future elders that might be useful to them and that might help them enhance their aging process and enable them to make a success of their elder role? What can society do to enhance the status and the well-being of future elders?

THE PERSONAL APPROACH TO AGING

Throughout this book we have considered toxic and nourishing ethical aspects of aging. We have learned that some persons approach old age with life-enhancing attitudes that reflect patterns developed throughout a lifetime. What guidelines can be drawn from these persons' lives that will suggest ways to age successfully, triumphantly without bitterness, anger, or unhealthy responses? The following suggestions may prove useful:

1. Recognize that "old age" is not a stage separated from the rest of life. It is part of a process or a continuum, and an extension of earlier life activities. Those who live a rich, healthy, full life throughout their earlier years have a better chance of enjoying a full, healthy old age.

2. Recognize yourself not as a "victim" of aging or as an innocent bystander in the life process, but as a source of that which is the make-up of your life. You decide whether your life will be nourishing, warm, and life-enhancing or toxic, cold, and life-denying.

3. Focus on your potential and talents rather than on losses, weaknesses, and problems. You are personally involved in determining the quality and direction of your life.

4. Don't brood over mistakes; instead, learn from them and move on. View life as a great teacher and take advantage of the rich potentials it offers. Learn from the past, be involved in the present, contribute to the future.

5. Choose role models you can look to and admire; select persons who are examples of successful living and successful aging. Explore biographies and autobiographies for insights and episodes, events and ideas that gave quality to the life of these role models.

6. Look about you and see what kind of persons others are. Note the nourishing as well as the toxic elements in their lives, then emulate the former and avoid the latter.

7. Don't lay back and rest in positive thinking alone; take active steps to improve any situation you may be in.

8. Involve yourself in personal health care; maintain a health diet, exercise, avoid stress, have fun. There are so many choices. Some include swimming, bike-riding, walking, golf, yoga, meditation and other relaxation techniques. Work toward making your life healthier.

9. Continue to make new friends. When old friends move away or die, you will have the skills to move into new relationships with new acquaintances, friends, and lovers.

10. Be involved mentally no matter what your age. Explore academic courses in high schools, colleges, universities, churches, and senior residences. Some elders have become so involved in new educational adventures that they have moved into campus dormitories to mingle with younger students and keep in touch with how youth are reacting to the world around them.

11. Continue to work after retirement, if that interests you. But work because you like to be actively engaged. Many employers prefer elders because they are reliable, dependable, and oftentimes do a better job than their younger counterparts.

12. Get involved in volunteer service.

13. Avoid becoming a long-winded talker. Many elders learned to listen during their maturing periods, hence they listen and share rather than give advice and preach.

14. Discover the joys of giving, which can be more rewarding than receiving. Givers tend to avoid whining about their lot because they are involved with the needs of others.

15. Move out and into life. Avoid being cooped up in the house tied to television "soaps" and game shows. Often television addiction begins in childhood and continues on into maturity until it becomes a way of life. Live adventurously by travelling down different streets, taking bus trips or train trips, or, if possible, travel abroad. Enter into the adventure of discovering new places, new foods, new people.

16. Place greater emphasis on the little things in life that bring pleasure and far less on what "society" and what others find important. The greater the effort expended in moving away from toxic experiences and situations, the greater the energy available for expanding environments and the pursuit of nourishing qualities.

17. Learn to live in moments, not years. Few people recall the details of any particular year. They remember events, moments that occurred within a given time period. The particular year is of minor importance, it is the experience of the special moment that counts. Form a necklace of those moments that are somehow apart from the ordinary and mark high points in relationships, aesthetic experiences, or social activities, and then, through memory, continue to savor their exquisiteness.

18. Learn to love life. There is awesome wonder in nature: from the immensity of the cosmos to the tiniest organisms, from snow-capped mountains to the splendid farm lands and forests, lakes and seashores and into the intricate complexities of the huge cities. Love living and love life.

19. Discover the integrating experiences that change life, that give direction, that shape the course of subsequent events, and provide the insights by which we live. These happenings, which Abraham Maslow has described as "peak experiences," determine the self, bring wholeness, and reorganize life.

Some years ago, when I was about to leave Cairo, Egypt, I was fortunate in being driven to the airport by a very well-educated cab driver. As we were chatting, he suddenly stopped talking for a couple of moments, then apologized, explaining that he had prayed we were passing the cemetery where his father was entombed in the family burial vault. He told me that his father's death had produced a life-changing moment. He, the eldest son, had been in Lebanon when his father died, and because burials were made on the day of death, he had been unable to fulfill the funeral obligations of the first-born son. He visited all near relatives and received from them the promise that at the next death of a family member, he would be permitted to enter the mausoleum with the immediate family of the deceased so that he could pay his respects to his father.

After a three-month wait, a relative died and he went inside the mausoleum to be with his dead father. "What happened?" I asked. "I saw God!" he replied. "What my father was, I would become!" That experience so impacted on him that he changed his life pattern. "All my income is now divided into four parts. One part is set aside so I can take my mother on a pilgrimage to Mecca. One part goes to my wife for family needs. One part is saved so I can build up a fleet of taxis, and the last portion is spent with my wife and children in having fun together. My life with my family is all I have on earth before I go to join my father. What I do now has importance."

Consider what this man's peak experience did for him. It gave new direction and organization. He could harmonize the life-transforming event with insights that coincided with his Muslim faith to produce meaning and purpose. He reaffirmed his love for his aging mother and for his family. He expressed his responsibilities as a son, a father, a husband, and a wage-earner. He did not reject the work ethic but widened his interests to embrace enjoyment in life and the shared moments of his existence. He would build a business based on honesty, on good service, and the continuation of self-fulfillment.

Had he really changed? In some dimensions of his life, yes; in others, no. He had always been supportive of his family. He had helped one brother graduate from medical school and another become an engineer. But the focus of his life was now different; now it was on the awareness of the brevity of life, on what he could do for and with his family and how he could satisfy the inner man.

One of my own experiences was quite different. I was part of a team excavating the mound of the ancient city of Hebron, which is now in Israel, but was at that time in Jordan. I turn now to my records of that experience:

An excavator need not open many tombs or dig through many occupation levels before reflecting on the swift passage of life, on death and its causes. Sometimes the awareness of the brevity of human existence comes dramatically.

It was 5.00 A.M. on a beautiful morning in August. The grey sky was beginning to turn blue and the rising sun fringed the scattered clouds with gold and various hues of pink. A few crickets chirped in the old olive trees and the awakening birds began their morning songs. Suddenly, the serenity of those moments was pierced by a woman's keening wail that prickled the hair on my neck. Then another woman's voice, deeper in pitch but anguished and sob-filled, joined the first voice and the mingled cries seemed to cling to the ancient stone walls near which we were digging.

"What was that?" I asked. My teenaged Arab helper, Damon, solemnly replied, "She lost her man." During the night, the young father had died. The first voice belonged to his wife, the second to his mother. Throughout the early morning we heard them crying. Later we watched as the body was borne on a simple pallet to the mosque for prayers before internment in the family crypt.

We had just excavated the bones of a little child who had died beneath the massive rock from the ancient wall which had tumbled down during an earthquake a hundred years earlier in the nineteenth century. Lower on the slope some of our students were working in a cave-dwelling whose occupants had perished when part of the roof had collapsed about 3000 B.C.E. A few hundred yards away was a Byzantine cemetery where members of the Christian community had buried their dead during the sixth century C.E. and where one of our young students was supervising the excavation of several skeletons. Under such circumstances how could one fail to ponder the issues of life and death? The women's cries became symbols of the wailing of mothers and wives and of fathers, brothers, sisters, sons, and daughters at the death of loved ones—everywhere—throughout human history. Some died accidentally, some through pestilence and disease, but how many through man's callous treatment of man—through war, tyranny, hatred?

Here are the bones of past generations. Here are the household items used by families who occupied the houses whose foundations we have been clearing. Here are the little treasures of bronze, glass, and clay that were dear to them and which beautified and enhanced their lives—testimonies to man's creative genius. But how quickly life passes, and how unimportant are the "things" of life and how important are the moments that give meaning to individual existence.

How, then, shall I live in the light of the past?

Two phrases have burned themselves into my consciousness: one from a bookplate in a small volume that I purchased many years ago from a rabbi's library, the other from a delightful French film titled *The Shameless Old Lady*. The bookplate depicted a strong angelic figure standing on top of the world with the winds of space blowing against his garments. Above his head, he held a banner that read, "Better to burn out than to rust out." The last line in the film was "She ate of the bread of life and savored it to the last crumb."

As an archaeologist and historian, keenly conscious of how brief my few years are in the registry of thousands of years of human development, these sentences or slogans together with the experiences of this excavation at Hebron, prompt me to seek to press out of each moment all that I can of love, joy, peace, and pleasure to the extent that I might experience to the full the great and wonderful gift of life. This zest for and love of life relates to what I love doing most—working with people in ideas and artifacts that enable us to appreciate the marvelous history of man; to teaching and the encounter with students; to research and the probing of the past for the understanding of the future.

That was my experience as recorded over twenty-five years ago. As I look back over this past quarter century there can be no doubt that much of what I experienced then has motivated me, and continues to do so. But there have been other such moments with new experiences that have provided deepening insights and have caught me up in different and expanded concerns, including geroethics. The point I am trying to make through these examples is that into every life there come encounters that transform it, that provide wisdom or insight or guidance or direction, that integrate the self and that enable the person to discover who or what he or she is. We all have these experiences and each one transforms or shifts the person to some degree, one way or another. Sometimes the event is dramatic, as it was for the Cairo cab driver; at other times it can be a more reflexive harmonizing of a series of experiences as it was for me so many years ago. What is important is that we recognize these peak moments for what they are and ponder the ways in which they give direction to our lives.

BEYOND THE PERSONAL

It is obvious that geroethics must move beyond interest in personal ethical behavior and growth to embrace the whole of society. The United States has stalled far too long in developing a national health program. The number of elders and their families who have been damaged and stifled in growth and in well-being because of this failure cannot be estimated. Medicare and Medicaid are not enough. A simpler, more inclusive, less complicated, and more direct health-aid program must be brought about —and soon. Each year of delay handicaps thousands of citizens and promises even more ill and ailing persons, including elders, in the future. Elders and their families must exert pressure on their representatives in government to introduce a national health insurance program of a stature and quality. America should be a trend setter and an example to the world, rather than a follower with a very poor track record.

It is also time to publicize the need for elder protection against abuse of any kind. Just as places of refuge have been established for battered children and spouses, so, too, places of refuge should be available for battered elders. Nursing homes cannot be the answer, for they are not equipped to provide the counseling and succor needed. The evidence of maltreatment of elders needs to be publicly condemned, whether it results from financial duping or physical and psychological mistreatment. Elders need to be informed of their rights and of places where help can be found. Investigation of abuse and prosecution of abusers needs to be thorough and rapid. Only broad social awareness will result in change.

Research into the causes of aging and related illnesses needs funding. For some special-interest groups to thwart investigation of research that gives promise of slowing or eliminating certain diseases is both unethical and unfair. Our government needs to represent the best interests of elders, not the arguments of special-interest groups.

Elder needs will multiply, as the number of elders increases. Only as government officials are made conscious of their needs and persuaded to plan for the elders of the future will changes be made. We have made wonderful strides in some areas of elder care; the time for even greater progress is at hand.

GEROETHICS AND GLOBAL AGING

Up to this point, we have focussed on present gerontological issues but always with an eye to the future. Our emphasis has been on facets of aging in the First World, particularly America, but a global perspective has always been in the back of our mind. With regard to the future of those who live and are aging in poor Third-World countries, it is impossible to make predictions. At the present time they face frightening problems, including over-population, near starvation, and rampant disease. Many of the children who will mature into adulthood will be severely impaired by the effects of lack of food and proper medications. How many will enter old age cannot be estimated. Yet we in the First World dare not become insular in our thinking or in our concerns because the generation of those of us who are today's elders have called forth changes in perspective that cannot be ignored.

For example, modern archaeology and paleontology have informed us that through DNA studies it has been demonstrated that we, as a human species, may truly be one family, having evolved from a single mother (interestingly enough called "Eve" or "Eva") who, millennia ago, lived in Africa. This suggests that our concerns for one another must be familial, bridging racial, ethnic, territorial, and all other gaps that today separate us. We must be involved in the struggle to gain that new tomorrow when the importance of our oneness will be more significant than the social structures that presently tend to separate us. To be truly concerned about geroethics for the future, we must be concerned for aging patterns affecting the well-being of all members of our human family.

Space exploration has provided us with photographs of planet earth. We have been made aware that, for better or for worse, we are all members of one global household. Therefore, whatever happens in one section of our dwelling place affects and has implications for the whole. When large industries pour toxic wastes into central water systems like the Rhine River in Europe; when large corporations deplete forests in North America and rain forests in South America for profit; when an Iraqi tyrant fouls water and air with spilled and burning oil; when food sent to starving people in Ethiopia is held up and not delivered; when a Rumanian tyrant insists on the breeding of children and then confines them in intolerable and inhumane institutional settings; when a nuclear explosion occurs in Chernobyl, Russia; and when chemical leaks impact on a town in India, then, because the world is my home, my anger, my frustration, and my fear grows. I am angry and frustrated because of my helplessness to somehow intervene personally and make changes, and I fear for the future of my (and our) great grandchildren, whom I (we) will never see but who will be affected by what this, my generation of elders, is doing and has done. To be sure, I can and do support organizations that seek to curb and correct these terrible happenings, always trying to be careful to select those who actually use financial donations for the projects in which they claim to be involved rather than syphoning off 90 percent or more for their own salaries and advertising; always trying to determine whether or not the organization has a hidden purpose such as using food and care of children to evangelize and spread their own narrow faith system. I choose to be an ethically involved elder, but my single efforts seem so small and my voice appears to be lost in the din of the larger impersonal world.

Like other ethical elders, I am naturally concerned with events, policies, and programs that affect the well-being and the health of those in my own bailiwick. But this is not enough. That worldview is too small, too limited. We elders have moved beyond the world we inherited sixty-five and more years ago and have been instrumental in developing global awareness. With that awareness comes global responsibility for ourselves and for the future. What does this imply?

Every elder who is genuinely concerned with geroethics needs to have a small globe or picture of the planet earth nearby on a table or pinned to the wall to keep him or her aware of our cosmic setting. Every elder needs to become part of the action to transform the world into a co-operating household of family members—the awareness of which his or her generation has produced.

The residue of our having been here, alive, on planet earth needs to be more than a casket of dried bones in a cemetery or a handful of ashes buried or scattered. The residue must be the impact, however small, of our presence expressed in genuine concern for the future of the species and of the planet. Our efforts may be limited, but they can be real— as simple as planting a tree to help produce better air quality, picking up and depositing the trash left by careless others, recycling our household refuse, writing letters to the press or to our political representatives concerning key social issues, or by supporting a cause or a candidate seeking the betterment of humankind. Or our effort can be as grand as endowing a chair (in Gerontology?) in a university or providing a wing to a hospital, building a center for research, or underwriting a cause. Every positive and nourishing act counts as a contribution to a better future and to leaving the world a better place than it was when we first entered it. Our society has grown in complexity and every human service makes its own unique contribution. As a part of that society, we either seek to exploit, use, and disregard the rights of others (both the living and those who will form later generations) or we live to fulfill our own lives and the lives of others, seeking the health and well-being of humans everywhere— both now and in the future. These are the ethical choices. What we do now constitutes, in part, our gift to the future and to some degree determines the shape of that future. We are not a group of helpless, doddering old fogies; we are alive and we can be socially and ethically involved, demanding our rights and our recognition as significant humans who seek to bring about changes that will transform this troubled world into a place that is just a bit closer to the highest dreams and ideals envisioned by sensitive and caring humans. It matters now that we are here; it can matter to the future that we have been here.

REFERENCE

Montagu, Ashley. 1960. "Problems of an Aging Population," *Journal of the National Medical Association* 52, pp. 338–42 (reprinted in Ashley Montagu, *The Humanization of Man,* Cleveland, Ohio: The World Publishing Company, 1962, pp. 247–56).